The Art of *Aromatherapy*

The Healing and Beautifying Properties
of the Essential Oils of Flowers and Herbs

Christine S. Negm, MS, RD
30 Plaza Way #4
Chico, CA 95926-1237

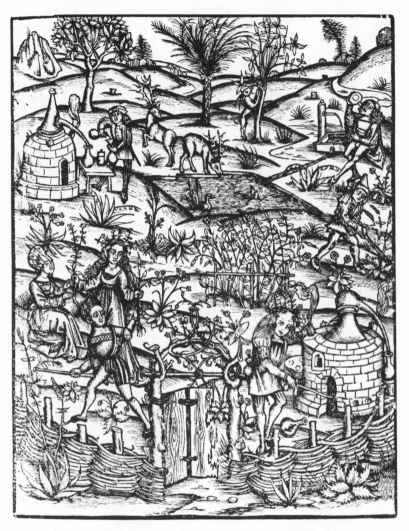

'Spare not favourable reder to pursue and revolve to thy synguler helthe, conforte, and lernynge, this booke of dystyllacyon. Lerne the hygh and mervelous vertue of herbes, knowe how inestimable a preservatyve to the helth of man god hath provyded growyng every daye at our hande, use the effectes with reverence, and give thankes to the maker celestyall.'

Laurens Andrewe, *The Vertuose Boke of Distyllacyon of the Waters of all Maner of Herbes* by Hieronymus Braunschweig, (1527).

The Art of
Aromatherapy

The Healing and Beautifying Properties
of the Essential Oils of Flowers and Herbs

New Revised Edition

Robert B. Tisserand

HEALING ARTS PRESS
Rochester, Vermont

Healing Arts Press
1 Park Street
Rochester, VT 05767

First published in Great Britain by The C. W. Daniel
Company Ltd., Essex. England.

Library of Congress Cataloging in Publication Data

Tisserand, Robert.
 The art of aromatherapy.

 Bibliography: p.
 1   Essences and essential oils–Therapeutic use.
2.   Aromatic plants–Therapeutic use.   I.   Title.
RS164. T57 -1978   615'.3   77-20493
ISBN 0-89281-001-7

Healing Arts Press is a division of Inner Traditions International.

Printed in the United States of America.

15

Foreword

'My father took down some bottles from over the fireplace and mixed several liquids in a bowl. He then made a compress by folding a small piece of flannel, soaked it in the liquid and placed it on the man's side. Within half an hour the pains had gone and his face was no longer screwed up out of all recognition as it had been. Gripping the table in my excitement I couldn't take my eyes off him: it was a miracle!

' "Papa, did *you* do that!"

' "Mon chéri, he who causes the plants to grow is the one who did it." '

Of Men and Plants
Maurice Mességué

At one time there was no distinction between science and art, between knowledge and ability. A man could be barber, dentist, surgeon, and herbalist all in one; or he could be a great painter, philosopher, and mathematician. The old apothecary was the equivalent of a combination of modern herbalist and pharmacist. As the sixteenth and seventeenth centuries went by he became less and less of a herbalist and, by degrees, more of a pharmacist.

As we have split knowledge into art and science, science has become more powerful, more predominant. At first sight it seems practical, and indeed is, to have telephones, computers, televisions, and so on. But, like a child with a new toy, we misuse our abilities; we do not know how to restrain or control such things, or put them to the uses for which they were created. Instead they become instruments with which to spread suffering — war, political bias, economic disaster.

The word 'knowledge' itself has narrowed in its meaning. It now means something you know — a fact, or collection of facts. It does not imply any practical ability at all. We have arrived at the point where money, power, and scientific fact have become ends in themselves, instead of being means to bring about a more comfortable, peaceful, and happy life. Our minds have run away with us, and as we have become obsessive, so we have become steadily more neurotic. As doctors increase their knowledge of disease so disease becomes more tenacious and widespread. As new drugs are formulated and marketed, the harm done by such drugs increases proportionately.

In recent years there has been, or begun, a backlash against this trend. Such arts as astrology, acupuncture, and organic farming have been the recipients of a tremendous surge of interest. The word 'natural' has become the central core of a great deal of advertising, and natural food (what other kind of food can there be?) has boomed.

We went too far in one direction, and we are just beginning to redress the balance. It is a natural process, and as inevitable as the swing of a pendulum. It seems, however, that the only way to stop the pendulum swinging like a gigantic scythe across the world, cutting back and forth, is for each one of us to find the point of balance and stay there.

Thus, although this book concerns the aesthetic side of aromatherapy, and I myself incline to the intuitive mode of understanding, I have not neglected its scientific aspects. There has been considerable research on the medicinal properties of essences in recent years, and a revival of interest in the pharmaceutical possibilities of 'botanicals' in general. Medical science has long since grown out of the idea that *all* pharmaceutical preparations could be made synthetically, and without the use of plants and plant extracts. Along with the trend 'back to nature' we find that pharmacists are looking for new drugs in forests and fields, as well as test-tubes.

The herbalists of previous centuries had a deep love of nature and respect for plants, and in some ways seemed to understand them better than we do today. They knew where to find their plants growing naturally. They knew in which season and at what time of day to pick them; which planets ruled them, and how this affected their properties. They knew virtually nothing of the chemical constituents of the herbs, or why they had certain properties. But they knew a little about disease, and knew which herbs were good for certain ailments. This knowledge was based on no kind of science, except that of trial and error, added to the experience of their predecessors and, perhaps more significantly, their own intuition.

It was their intuition or inspiration which led them successfully to combine astrology with herbal medicine, and which led to the formation of the doctrine of signatures. Because their knowledge was based almost entirely on experience it was (and still is) a more practical knowledge than that of scientific experiment and trial. So often a drug is marketed only to be withdrawn years later, because it has been found to be unsafe; the same is true of food additives. The test of time is still the ultimate test and natural medicines, like natural foods, are the only safe ones.

When I began researching this book I decided to consult as many and varied sources as possible — from perfumery books to pharmacopoeias, from the USA to China, from the earliest manuscripts up to the latest scientific findings. This, as I soon realised, would be the task of a lifetime, but I have, I hope, taken a fair account of each type of literature. I am greatly indebted to the works of Dr Valnet (whose book *Aromathérapie* first introduced me to the subject) as I am to the works of Professor Rovesti, and the many other books and articles consulted.

Aromatherapy is a subject which, at least in England, has so far been steeped in magic and mystery. This may give it a certain amount of appeal, but it also creates a great deal of confusion and misunderstanding, and leaves most people in a state of relative ignorance. I hope that this book will help to shed some light on the subject.

What therefore is aromatherapy? Is it no more than a branch of herbal medicine? In the sense that it is an attempt to heal through medicines of botanical origin, this statement is true, but there the comparison ends. In fact the use of essential oils is not taught by the National Institute of Medical Herbalists (one of the best herbal schools in the world), neither are essences used by the majority of herbalists. Also, herbal medicine is based on the

7

organic principle of using the whole herb, or its extract, and essential oils hardly fit into this category.

Essences are like the blood of a person. They are not the whole plant, but are whole, organic substances in themselves. Like blood they will die (lose their life force) if they are not properly preserved. Like blood they incorporate the characteristics of the body (plant) from which they come. They are like the personality, or spirit, of the plant. The essence is the most ethereal and subtle part of the plant, and its therapeutic action takes place on a higher, more subtle level than that of the whole, organic plant, or its extract, having in general a much more pronounced effect on the mind and emotions than herbal medicine. The properties of herbs and their essences may be much the same, but the therapeutic action itself is different.

Aromatherapy is unusual in that its remedies may be applied either externally or internally when treating internal disorders. In the words of René-Maurice Gattefossé, the pioneer of modern aromatherapy: 'The products are externally applied, but their penetrative power is sufficiently great for them to act on the organs subjacent to the areas to which the topical applications are made.' The brain, the nervous system, and the sense organs are all derived from the ectoderm of the embryo at the same time as the skin. Their common origin means that they maintain very close connections throughout life, and it is reasonable to assume that products applied to an area of skin affect the subjacent organs, even if no penetration were to take place. This association is reflected in Hilton's Law, which states that the nerve which supplies a joint also supplies the muscles which move the joint, and the skin over the joint.

This is a personal book. I have seldom hesitated to express my opinion, although I naturally do not expect everyone to agree with everything I say. Although the given properties of the essences are largely based on scientific research, they should not all be taken as proved. This book is not intended as a medical textbook. Anyone who is seriously ill should consult a qualified medical practitioner. Although I am a strong believer in natural healing, I know of cases where people have hurt themselves or others because of insufficient knowledge.

Aromatherapy cannot be divorced from a number of things: the basic principles of natural therapeutics, massage, diet, and our whole attitude to life. This is why many pages are devoted to these same subjects. The boundaries of any subject are simply where you put them, and it is difficult to talk about anything without touching on related subjects.

Shapes relate to colour, to odours, tastes, moods, elements, organs, plants, diseases; everything interrelates. Of course, the analogies are never perfect but they enable us to see the order of the universe, the correlation between things which are apparently unconnected. What we are really talking about here is qualities, or vibrations. How do you know if two things have the same quality, or vibration? Only by feeling, by using that sixth sense which we call intuition. The more we develop our intuition the more we will be able to see the order and perfection of the universe, and the deeper and richer our lives will become.

Contents

Introduction to revised edition

It was in 1975 when I first started work on this book almost exactly ten years ago. Those ten years have seen a tremendous increase in the awareness, and popularity of aromatherapy, and it is now accepted as a form of 'alternative' medicine. During this period, with every magazine or newspaper article on aromatherapy, with every radio or television interview, and with the appearance of other books on the same subject. *The Art of Aromatherapy* has grown more and more in stature.

The book has also grown in another sense — it has become international. The first translation to appear was the German one, closely followed by editions in Italian, Spanish, Dutch and, most recently, Japanese. A separate edition is also published in the USA. The English edition alone has sold more than 20,000 copies.

Although there is no doubt that this book has played a very significant role in the emergence and development of aromatherapy in recent years, this event is, in turn, part of a broader trend towards fitness, health foods, and natural therapeutics.

So many people are now turning to 'alternative' forms of treatment, and one possible danger is that, almost blinded by the light of their new-found faith in all things natural, they will expect miracle cures: not miracle cures resulting from the doctor's prescription pad, but from the acupuncture needle, or the essential oil. Natural therapeutics as a whole are not, and never can be, based on 'magic bullets'; on natural wonder drugs. A body which has been ravaged for years by alcohol or tobacco, by junk food or anxiety, by overwork or neglect will simply not be capable of responding overnight to any kind of natural remedy. True healing takes time, and it also requires understanding and co-operation on the part of the patient.

There are two points which I would like to make very clear:

Firstly, essential oils are already used as home remedies by thousands of people, and I can see no harm in this *provided that the oils are sensibly and correctly used*. I believe that we should all take a more informed interest in our own health, and for this reason I hold a one-day seminar for the lay person (see page 320). Essential oils can be fun to use as room fresheners, in the bath, or in massage, and they can be extremely useful as home remedies for many of the more minor ailments.

Secondly, we must realise that self-treatment, although it has its place, also has its limitations. Do treat yourself for simple, common ailments, but for any long-term, or deep-seated problem, seek professional advice. This book is not intended as a self-treatment handbook for such ailments as dysentery, cancer or tuberculosis. If in doubt consult your health practitioner.

Aromatherapy is practised in quite different ways by different groups of people, including doctors (in France there are literally hundreds of general practitioners who have trained in aromatherapy) psycho-therapists, beauty therapists, massage therapists, aromatherapists and lay people. In attempting to write a book which speaks to all of you I run the risk of either boring the more serious therapist, or losing the lay person in a mass of technical jargon. Inevitably some sections of the book will be more readable, or more interesting to you than others.

Aromatherapy is very versatile; not only do we use the oils in a variety of ways, taking them by mouth, using them in massage, inhalations, baths and so on; but the oils themselves work on three distinct levels. In the literal sense of the word 'aromatherapy' the aromas play an important role. Call it psychosomatic, but they do make us *feel* better, and *feeling* better can have a tremendous therapeutic influence on physical symptoms. So much physical illness is in fact, to some degree, stress-related.

Aromatherapy is not only psychosomatic. The oils all work on the physical body in a variety of ways, and they are among the most potent anti-bacterial agents known to man. They certainly present an interesting, and viable alternative to anti-biotic drugs.

Essential oils can also be used to 'balance' the subtle energy flows in the body, in a similar way to acupuncture. This is something which I have been researching in recent years, and it forms a significant part of the aromatherapy courses which I am now teaching (see page 320).

In this new, revised edition Pennyroyal essential oil has been excluded for safety reasons, the 'Recipe' section has been improved and made more readable, and a large number of alterations and additions have been made.

I have watched this book develop as one watches a child grow — with patience mingled with frustration, but, overall, with a sense of pride and wonder. My hope is that it will help to broaden your own horizon just a little.

Robert Tisserand
January 1985

Chapter 1

About Essential Oils

'God of his infinite goodnesse and bounty hath by
the medium of Plants, bestowed almost all food,
clothing and medicine upon man.'

Gerarde's *Herbal* (1636)

Aromatic oils are used in three classes of consumer goods:
foods, toiletries, and medicines. In foods they are used as
natural flavourings, such as oils of lemon, orange, and lime in
marmalades. In cosmetics they are incorporated both in perfumes and, less often, as natural active ingredients; they are also
widely used in toothpaste flavourings. In medicine they are used
not only as flavouring agents but as therapeutic ingredients in
their own right. The use of clove oil for toothache, peppermint
oil for indigestion, and eucalyptus for inhalations is well
known. Essences are also used in a number of patented medicinal products, including antiseptic creams and ointments, inhalations (such as friar's balsam), hair tonics (bay rum), ointments
for skin diseases, rubefacient liniment for rheumatic pain, and
so on. Primarily they are included in preparations for external
application, although recently a UK patent was taken out for a
gallstone-dissolving product which contains a number of essences.

Essential oils are odorous and highly volatile (they readily
evaporate in the open air). They are quite different from fatty
oils, and have a consistency more like water than oil. Their
chemistry is complex, but they generally contain alcohols,
esters, ketones, aldehydes, and terpenes. The odoriferous
materials are formed in the chloroplasts of the leaf. Here they
combine with glucose to form glucosides, which are transported

around the plant structures.

Most essences are clear, although a few (especially the absolutes) are coloured, some being red (benzoin), others green (bergamot), yellow (lemon), or blue (camomile). They are soluble in alcohol, ether, and fixed oils, but insoluble in water.

The oils are present in tiny droplets in a large number of plants, especially those most commonly used for their culinary and medicinal properties. They can occur in roots (calamus), leaves (rosemary), flowers (lavender), barks (cinnamon), resins (myrrh) and the rind of some fruits. The presence of essential oil in oranges can be demonstrated by squeezing a section of the peel next to a lighted match: the oil droplets will spray out and briefly ignite as they pass through the flame. The scent of flowers and herbs is due to their essential oil content, as is the spiciness of spices.

Essences are usually extracted by distillation. This involves placing the plant material in a vat and passing steam through it. The essences evaporate along with water and other substances. The distillate is then cooled, and the essences (which are not water-soluble) are easily separated from the water. Sometimes other methods are favoured, the most common alternative being extraction by volatile solvents. The plant material (usually flowers) is washed in a suitable solvent, such as alcohol, until the essence is dissolved in the solvent. It is then separated by being distilled at a precise temperature which condenses the oil but not the solvent: the oil thus obtained is known as an 'absolute'.

Yet another method, which is usually employed for citrus fruits, is carried out completely by hand. The peel is cut off from the pulp, and then squeezed over a bucket, which collects the oil along with a little juice. This has now been largely superceded by mechanised pressing, and distillation is also sometimes used.

While they are in the plant the essences are constantly changing their chemical composition, and move from one part of the plant to another according to the time of day and the seasons. This is why plants destined for oil extraction must be picked at a certain time of year, in certain weather conditions, and usually at a certain time of day. The odour and chemical constituents of essences change with different soil conditions, variations in climate, and methods of cultivation. This is why oils from certain countries, like Bulgarian Rose and Ceylonese cinnamon, are considered to be of a higher quality than those from other countries.

The amount of essence present in the plant varies from about 0.01% up to 10% or even more. Rose petals, for instance, contain very little essence, and up to 2,000 kg of petals may be needed to produce 1 kg of oil.

Some oils, like those from rose, jasmine, carnation, and tuberose, are particularly heavy and concentrated. These are known as absolutes, and because they are so concentrated (and so expensive) very little is needed. Some essences, such as Bulgarian rose otto, are solid at room temperature and need to be warmed before they assume the usual fluidity of essences.

The effects of heat, light, air, and moisture generally have a damaging effect on essential oils. They should therefore always be kept in dark, airtight bottles and in cool, dry conditions.

There are hundreds of aromatic plants, only some of which are used to produced essences commercially. About a third of the plants traditionally used in herbal medicine are aromatic. No two of them smell exactly alike, and the properties of each are unique. The essence of a plant is like its personality. All animals, including humans, have their own characteristic smell, quite apart from what we call body odour. We are not commonly aware of our own scent, nor usually of other people's. We may, however, perceive it on a subconscious level, and it may influence our feeling towards each other more than we realise.

There is little doubt that scent has some practical use in the plant kingdom. Animals (and probably humans) are sexually attracted by aromatic substances called pheromones. It is suggested by Peter Tompkins and Christopher Bird in their book *The Secret Life of Plants* that essences have a similar role:

> 'Flowers that remain unfertilized emit a strong fragrance for as many as eight days or until the flower withers and falls; yet once impregnated the flower ceases to exude its fragrance, usually in less than half an hour.'

This idea places plants in a more sexual or animal light than has so far been generally accepted. Nevertheless, there are plants which exhibit other animal traits, such as carnivorous plants, which eat insects. A more commonly accepted idea is that the scent of a plant attracts certain insects which, by moving from plant to plant, cause fertilisation to take place. Essential oils are in fact used commercially to attract or repel certain insects. The essences of many plants are a natural defence mechanism, repelling insects which would otherwise harm the plant.

It has also been said of essences that they are mere waste products of plant metabolism. Surely if its use becomes known it ceases to be a mere waste product? I find it hard to believe that essences, which are in general highly complex and pleasant substances, are merely waste products. I prefer to believe that aromatic plants were created for man to use and enjoy, as perfumes and as medicines, and that the aromatic principle also serves as an aid to plant fertilisation. After all, is it merely coincidence that we find flowers pleasing to look at and to smell?

A Russian article on the physiological role of essential oils in plants revealed, in 1965, the results of a study on caraway, juniper, and coriander. It indicates that essential oils are not merely plant secretions, but rather that they 'actively participate in the development of plants'. The evaporation of essences from the plant surface is seen as a defence mechanism against infection by bacteria, fungi, and pests. Aromatic plants have a protective aura of scent, just as all living things have an aura of light. This aromatic aura also protects plants from excesses of heat and cold.

> 'From inside comes the voice and from inside comes the scent. Just as one can tell human beings in the dark from the tone of voices, so in the dark, every flower can be recognised by its scent. Each carries the soul of its progenitor.'

The above lines were written by a nineteenth-century German doctor, Gustav Fechner. He was a man of great spiritual insight, and could see the auras of plants. It seemed to him that 'plant people', calmly living their lives in one spot, might well wonder why we humans were so keen on rushing about. He wrote:

> 'In addition to souls which run and shriek and devour, might there not be souls which bloom in stillness, exhale fragrance and satisfy their thirst with dew and their impulses by their burgeoning?'

Could not flowers, Fechner asked, communicate with each other by the very perfumes they exude, becoming aware of each other's presence in a way more delightful than by means of the verbiage of humans which is seldom delicate or fragrant except, by coincidence, in lovers?

Chapter 2

From Ancient Times

'Excellent herbs had our fathers of old,
Excellent herbs to ease their pain,
Alexanders and Marigold,
Eyebright, Orris, and Elecampane.'

Rudyard Kipling

Our distant ancestors, tens of thousands of years ago, must have known how and what to eat before they even knew how to make fire and cook food. Even in those early times they may have known simply from experience that some plants were poisonous, some would induce vomiting or diarrhoea, and others aided digestion. They almost certainly used their nose, as well as their eyes, to determine whether a plant was the one they were seeking, or whether it was suitable to eat.

It is impossible to point to a date when plants were first used medicinally. In the course of thousands of years the healing virtues of plants must have gradually been discovered. When man learned how to make fire he must have sometimes burned aromatic plants, finding that some were good to eat with cooked food, and that others made a pleasant smell. Not having aromatic gum trees in Europe, our ancestors probably used rosemary and thyme for their incense.

Through burning aromatic plants they would have discovered other properties; sometimes the smoke would be 'good to breathe', sometimes it would make one feel drowsy or invigorated. ('Smoking' a patient is one of the earliest recorded forms of treatment with herbs; it was often used to drive out evil spirits.) These plants also came to be used for other reasons, perhaps being burnt as offerings to the sun or Mother Earth, or on the birth of a child or the death of an enemy. Noticing the effects of herbal infusions and decoctions on the body, and the effects of 'herb smoke' on the mind, early man naturally attributed some power to them. As offerings, then, they had a real significance, and were associated with the earliest forms of ritual and magic. Even today, in some parts of the world, herbs are only picked when the moon and stars are in certain positions, and a particular chant is recited as the plant is being gathered, sometimes a different chant being required for each herb.

The senses of our distant ancestors were probably more acute than ours. Civilisation may bring refinement in some senses, but it cannot increase the acuity of our basic instincts and the perception of our senses. We do not use our nose to 'smell' the direction of the wind, the whereabouts of an enemy, or the tracks of an animal, although there are a few tribes in South America who can track by smell. Smelling fine perfumes may increase our appreciation of sophisticated scents, but we have lost the ability to smell an enemy, a poisonous herb, or a particular disease. It has been said before that the sense of smell is very closely linked to the proverbial 'sixth sense'.

During the neolithic period of the Eastern world, between 6,000 and 9,000 years ago, man discovered that plants such as olive, castor, and sesame contained fatty oil, which could be extracted by pressing. The flax plant, which was also used to make clothes, yielded linseed oil. If, at this period, man could bake bread and use herbs in cooking and in medicine, it is quite plausible to suppose that he could make scented oils. He undoubtedly used fatty oils to rub on his body and in his hair. Finding that these oils went rancid after a time and began to smell bad, it is possible that he began to scent them with the aromatic herbs commonly used in the kitchen, on the fire, and in medicines. If such scented oils were made by neolithic man, he may then have found that they had similar effects to the herbs, when the body was massaged with them.

A number of vessels, mostly made of alabaster and dating between 3000 and 2000 BC, can be seen in the Egyptian rooms of the British Museum. Some of them look uncommonly like ointment pots, and others, more vertically orientated, were probably made for scented oils. For the period in which they were living the Egyptian people were incredibly advanced; so much so, in fact, that the pyramids they built still present us with a number of un-solved questions which the most scientific mind cannot unravel. In the words of Eugene Rimmel:

> 'Whilst the Jews and other surrounding people were confined to the simplicities of pastoral life, the Eygp-tians were enjoying the luxuries of refinement, and car-ried them to an extent which was not surpassed, if equalled, by those who, after them, successively held the sceptre of civilization.'

How were their pyramids built? How were such enormous stones made to fit so perfectly together, to form an enormous, perfect shape containing hundreds of yards of tunnels and tombs? No satisfactory answer has yet been given. Perhaps we have found a clue to the reason for their shape, in the fact that it preserves corpses, whether they are embalmed or not. But if this is the reason, how did the Egyptians come to discover it?

If we look at their buildings, their carvings, their culture, and their art, we see a nation at the very height of civilisation. This is the same period in which one of the oldest books in the world is supposed to have been written. *The Yellow Emperor's Classic of Internal Medicine*, a Chinese text, was written by Huang Ti, the Yellow Emperor or Yellow Lord. This ancient author also knew things that we are only now beginning to understand. His book deals mainly with the causes and treatment of disease, and is the most important text for all acupuncturists, even the Chinese.

While the Chinese were developing acupuncture the Egyptians were, among other things, acquiring a knowledge of essences. The twelfth dynasty was the golden age of Egyptian jewellery; during this time cosmetics were also widely used. These consisted mainly of kohl (an early equivalent to our mascara) eyeshadow, which was usually green, and various unguents and ointments to beautify the complexion. They used red ochre to colour the lips and cheeks, and henna to stain the hands and fingernails a deep orange-yellow. White lead was also used to whiten the face, but being highly poisonous it was probably not much used. Some very beautiful cosmetic boxes have been recovered, dating from the twelfth dynasty (*c.* 2000 BC). These ornate boxes contain small pots and jars made of stone, which would have contained some of the cosmetics mentioned above, including scented unguents.

When the tomb of Tutankhamen was opened in 1922 a number

of such vases and scent pots were discovered, some containing unguents. These had been placed in the tomb when it was sealed in 1350 BC, over 3,000 years ago. The pots were made of calcite and the contents, which had solidified, later revealed the presence of frankincense, and something resembling Indian spikenard. These were mixed in a base of animal fat, which formed 90% of the mixture. The scent, though understandably faint, was still detectable.

At first these unguents were probably highly valued, and only used by royal families and perhaps the high priests. Later on they would become less sacred, and more widely used by ordinary people. They would be used in cosmetics, massage oils, medicines, and so on. There are papyri recording the medicinal use of herbs dating back to the reign of Khufu, who built the Great Pyramid around 2800 BC. All these records show that magic was considered to be just as effective as medicine: in order for a remedy to have its full effect it was customary for the physician to recite a magical formula four times. This kind of recitation was common in many other civilisations, and is still used by herbalists or witch doctors, in parts of Africa. An ancient Babylonian tablet has been found containing the following incantation for fever:

> 'The sick man . . . thou shalt place
> . . . thou shalt cover his face
> Burn cypress and herbs . . .
> That the great gods may remove the evil
> That the evil spirit may stand aside
> . . .
> May a kindly spirit, a kindly genius be present.'

The Ebers papyrus, dating from the eighteenth dynasty, shows that Egyptian physicians had a thorough knowledge of the properties of a large number of herbs. Here is a recipe for eye inflammation (translated from heiroglyphics):

> Myrrh
> 'Great Protectors' seed
> Copper oxide
> Lemon pips
> Northern cypress flowers
> Antimony
> Gazelle's droppings

Oryx offal
White oil

The directions for use are as follows:

'Place in water, let stand for one night, strain through a cloth, and smear over the eye for four days.'

Myrrh is still used today as an anti-inflammatory agent. Here is a recipe for a cosmetic face pack, from the same papyrus:

Ball of incense
Wax
Fresh oil
Cypress berries
'Crush, and rub down and put in new milk and apply it to the face for six days.'

The incense would refer to myrrh, or frankincense, or a mixture of the two. It was made into small balls for burning in a type of censer. This recipe bears an amazing resemblance to modern natural face packs. In another papyrus, written about 2000 BC, there is an account of the writer's journey into Nubia, in which he says:

'I will cause to be brought into thee fine oils and choice perfumes, and the incense of the temples, whereby every god is gladdened. Of myrrh hast thou not much; all that thou hast is but common incense. Ashipu came and delivered me, and he gave me a shipload of myrrh, fine oil, divers perfumes, eye-paint and the tails of giraffes.'

The first people to dispense aromatics were the priests; they were the first perfumers, the first aromatherapists. As the use of aromatics became more common they were also employed by physicians. The above recipes show a familiarity with the properties of aromatic gums, and suggest that they had been in use for some time already. At the base of the Sphinx at Giza there is a tablet of granite showing King Thutmos (1425 – 1408 BC) offering incense and libations of oil to a god with the body of a lion. Aromatics were also being widely used in medicines and cosmetic preparations at this time. The eighteenth dynasty, which began around 1580 BC, saw a considerable increase in wealth, trade, and power for Egypt; literature, art, painting, and sculpture flourished, and during this period the knowledge of aromatics increased considerably.

During the 1,500 years following the eighteenth dynasty the Egyptians perfected their knowledge of the medicinal properties of aromatics, of perfumery, and of the making of scented unguents and oils. There was not always a clear distinction between medicines and perfumes, and one item often served both purposes. Their preparations were kept in bottles, vases or pots made of alabaster, onyx, glass, or other hard substance, or sometimes in boxes made of carved wood or ivory. The aromatics used included myrrh, frankincense, cedarwood, origanum, bitter almond, spikenard, henna, juniper, coriander, calamus, and many other indigenous plants. Gradually a considerable international trade of gums and spices was built up. At Heliopolis, the City of the Sun, which was worshipped under the name of Ra, incense was burned three times a day: 'resin' was burned at sunrise, myrrh at noon, and a mixture of sixteen ingredients, called *kuphi*, or *kyphi*, at sunset. This last preparation was later used by both the Greeks and the Romans. The French chemist, Loret, has suggested that its chief constituents were calamus, cassia, cinnamon, peppermint, citronella, pistacia, *convulvulvus scoparius*, juniper, acacia, henna, cyperus, 'resin', myrrh, and raisins! Plutarch said of *kyphi* that it 'lulled one to sleep, allayed anxieties and brightened dreams'.

It has been widely recorded that the Egyptians used 'cedarwood oil' in the process of mummification. It is most likely that this was a pure essence extracted by pressing the wood, although it has been suggested that they used a primitive form of distillation, and some of the pots recovered from Egyptian tombs seem to support this theory; if this is true it means that distillation was known in Egypt at least 2,000 years before the Arabians were supposed to have invented it. Most of the other Egyptian oils, and certainly all those of the Greek and Roman periods, were infusions of aromatic herbs and gums in fatty oil. The fatty oil most widely used in Egypt was castor oil.

The Egyptians were not the only people to use aromatics at this period. There is a clay table from Babylon, dating from about 1800 BC, which is an order for 'imported oil of cedar, myrrh, and cypress'. This suggests that the knowledge of cedarwood oil extraction, and an international trade in aromatics, go back as much at 4,000 years. Cedarwood oil was highly prized both in Babylon and Egypt; it was used in oils and unguents for the hair and body, and was an ingredient in all the most expensive cosmetics. It was also used to smear over papyrus leaves to protect them from insects. The use of myrrh, cedarwood oil, and other aromatics in the process of mummification gives ample evidence of their antiseptic properties. The most well-preserved mummies are those which were most thoroughly embalmed with gums and spices. This has also led to the use of these gums as rejuvenating agents, to preserve the youthfulness of the skin. Great as was the consumption of perfumes in Egypt for religious rites and funerary honours, it was scarcely equal to the quantity of aromatics used for toilet purposes. One of the favourite ways to apply perfume, which was much used by Egyptian men, was to place a cone of solid unguent on the head; this would slowly melt, covering the head and body with perfume.

The Jewish peoples began their exodus from Egypt around 1240 BC, and their journey to the promised land took them some forty years. Shortly after they started Moses was given a number of commandments by the Lord, including how to make a holy oil and a holy incense:

> 'Moreover the Lord spake unto Moses, saying, Take thou also unto thee principal spices, of pure myrrh five hundred shekels, and of sweet cinnamon half so much, even two hundred and fifty shekels, and of sweet calamus two hundred and fifty shekels, And of cassia five hundred shekels, after the shekel of the sanctuary, and of oil olive an hin: And thou shalt make it an oil of holy anointment, an ointment compound after the art of the apothecary: it shall be an holy anointing oil' (Exodus 30, 22 – 25).

This oil was to be used only for holy purposes, and was not for common use among the people. However, we could not duplicate this recipe today even if we wanted to as there is much uncertainty and difference of opinion concerning the true botanical origin of the words 'myrrh' and 'calamus'; it seems likely that they do not refer to the plants which we now call by these names. The holy oil was used to consecrate Aaron and his sons, conferring on them perpetual priesthood from generation to generation. The ceremony was confined to the high priest and was performed by pouring oil on the head in sufficient quantity to run down on the beard and the skirts of the garments.

> 'And the Lord said unto Moses, Take unto thee sweet spices, stacte, and onycha, and galbanum; these sweet spices with pure frankincense: of each shall there be a like weight. And thou shalt make it a perfume, a confection after the art of the apothecary, tempered together, pure and holy.'

This perfume was also only for religious use; anyone disobeying this command would be 'cut off from his people'. The word 'perfume' is meant here in its original sense, from the Latin *per* (through) and *fumum* (smoke), that is to say incense. The true ingredients of this incense have also been lost to us, owing to the even greater confusion concerning the words 'stacte', 'onycha', and 'galbanum', although it is generally agreed that they all refer to aromatic gums.

The purification of Hebrew women took twelve months, the first six being accomplished by anointing regularly with 'oil of myrrh', which was probably an infused oil. Several aromatics were used for the second six months. As bathing was not always practical for Jewish women while they were trekking across the desert they developed the habit of wearing a small linen bag containing myhrrh and other aromatics. This was usually worn between the breasts, being hung from a cord around the neck, and constituted a long-lasting and effective deodorant.

The Song of Solomon contains much beautiful poetry, which often makes reference to aromatics:

> 'A bundle of myrrh is my well-beloved unto me; he shall lie all night betwixt my breasts. My beloved is unto me as a cluster of camphire in the vineyards of En-gedi . . .
>
> 'His cheeks are as a bed of spices, as sweet flowers: his lips like lilies, dropping sweet smelling myrrh . . .
>
> 'I am the rose of Sharon, and the lily of the valleys. As the lily among thorns, so is my love among the daughters . . .
>
> 'Thy plants are an orchard of pomegranates, with pleasant fruits; camphire, with spikenard; Spikenard and saffron; calamus and cinnamon, with all trees of

frankincense; myrrh and aloes, with all the chief
spices: A fountain of gardens, a well of living waters,
and streams from Lebanon.'

The Greeks learnt a great deal from the Egyptians concerning
perfumery, and the properties and uses of aromatics. Herodotus
and Democrates, who visited Egypt during the fourth century BC,
declared that the people were masters of the art of perfumery. It
was during this period that the Egyptians became familiar with
the art of floral extraction as depicted on the walls of the temple
of Edfu. This relief shows perfume being extracted from the
flowers of the white madonna lily, *Lilium candidum*, one of the
oldest plants still to be found in cottage gardens. It is not clear
whether this was a distillation of aromatic essence, or aromatic
water. Herodotus, who travelled widely, also mentions the
Assyrian women who would 'bruise with a stone wood of the
cypress, cedar and frankincense, and upon it poured water until it
became of a certain consistency. With this they anointed the body
and face to impart a most agreeable odour.' When removed on
the following day, it left the skin in a soft and beautiful condition
and impregnated with a delicious scent.

The Egyptians often ascribed the efficacy of aromatic medicines to the belief that they had been originally formulated, or
used, by one of the gods. The Greeks ascribed a divine origin to
all aromatic plants. In Greek mythology the invention of perfumes is attributed to the gods and, according to ancient belief,
men derived their knowledge of them from Aeone, a nymph of
Venus. Eugene Rimmel informs us that 'In those ancient times,
the only perfumes known appear to have been in the shape of oils
scented with flowers, and principally the rose'. Homer generally
designates them under the name of *elaion* (oil), adding sometimes
the epithet of 'rose' or 'ambrosial'. There is no mention of
distillation, and neither the Greeks nor, later, the Romans,
appear to have known of it. If the Egyptians did in fact know
how to distil essences, which seems improbable, they must have
kept this knowledge to themselves. Perhaps only a few high
priests actually knew the secret and, when Egypt came under
Roman rule, the knowledge died with them and remained buried
for nearly one thousand years.

The use of aromatic medicines and cosmetics was as prevalent
in Greece as in Egypt. The Greeks seemed to have been very

concerned about which part of the body to anoint with their scented concoctions. Diogenes always applied his unguents to his feet for, as he commented to those who mocked him for his eccentricity: 'When you anoint your head with perfume it flies away in the air, and birds only get the benefit of it; whilst if I rub it on my lower limbs it envelops my whole body, and gratefully ascends to my nose.' Anacreon, who was less concerned with the economics of the matter, recommended that the breast be anointed, as it was the seat of the heart (the emotional, as well as physical, heart). It was customary for the more wealthy Greeks to anoint different parts of the body with different scents; to quote Antiphanes:

> He bathes
> In a large gilded tub, and steeps his feet
> And legs in rich Egyptian unguent;
> His jaws and breasts he rubs with thick palm oil
> And both his arms with extract sweet, of mint;
> His eyebrows and his hair with marjoram,
> His knees and neck with essence of ground-thyme.'

The Greeks, the Romans, and all other 'perfumed' civilisations of antiquity, and indeed of more recent times, saw no fault in the male being as luxuriously perfumed as the female.

Many of the old perfumes were, as I have already indicated, also used for their medicinal properties. Since they were formulated entirely with natural ingredients they form a precise equivalent to modern aromatherapy products. One of the most famous Greek perfumes was called *megaleion*, after its creator, Megallus. As well as being used for its scent it was used to reduce skin inflammation and heal wounds. This is not surprising, since it contained a large amount of myrrh. Roy Genders tells us exactly how this produce was formulated:

> 'The oil of Balanos [a fatty oil] was boiled for ten
> days and nights to drive off impurities before the
> "burnt" resin was added. The myrrh was then pressed
> for several days, only the oily part known as "stakte"
> being used; and this was first mixed with cinnamon
> and cassia.'

The recipes for a number of medicinal perfumes are inscribed on marble tablets, both in the temples of Aesculapius, a Greek god of healing, and the temples of Aphrodite. According to legend Aesculapius, a child of Apollo and a nymph, was born at Epidauros, which later become a great city and health spa, with baths and healing centres. The healing essences were dispensed by priestesses, who succeeded the ancient magicians, and for a long time successfully competed with the products of ordinary perfumers and apothecaries. A Greek temple of aromatherapy!

One of the most celebrated cures effected at the spa, was of Milto, the young daughter of a humble Greek artisan. Every morning she would bring an offering to the temple of Aphrodite, in the form of a garland of fresh flowers; the poverty of her family prevented her from making a richer offering. She began to develop a tumour on her chin, which deeply saddened her, since she was a very beautiful young woman. One night, it is said, Aphrodite appeared to her in a dream, and told her to apply some of the roses from her altar to her chin. She did as the goddess instructed her, and recovered her beauty so completely that she eventually sat on the Persian throne as the favourite wife of Cyrus.

Marestheus, a renowned Greek physician, recognised that aromatic plants, especially flowers, usually had either stimulating or sedative properties. He mentions rose and hyacinth as being refreshing, invigorating a tired mind; most flowers with fruity or spicy scents having similar properties. The lily and narcissus, on the other hand, are more oppressive, causing stupor if their perfume is inhaled in sufficient quantity. Theophrastus believed that the scent of flowers was contained near the surface of the petals, and was released by the warmth of the sun; the scent of roots was released only by the warmth of the body or, as with incense, by fire. He recommended the use of olive oil to absorb the perfume of flowers; not only for its purity, but because the scent was so long-lasting when absorbed in oil or fat. Theophrastus wrote:

> 'It is to be expected that perfumes should have medicinal properties in view of the virtues of their spices. The effect of plasters and of what some call poultices prove these virtues, since they disperse tumours and abscesses and produce a distinct effect on the body and also its interior parts. If one lays a plaster on his abdomen and breast, he produces fragrant odours in his breath.'

27

The name of Cleopatra is legendary, and is inextricably linked with perfumery. She was the last of the Egyptian queens, although not of pure Egyptian blood. The old manufacturing art of perfumes and cosmetics had continued to develop in Egypt up till the time of Cleopatra, although by then being passed its climax. She, more Greek than Egyptian, ruled a dying empire; the force of her personality was sufficient to subdue Julius Caesar, as well as Mark Antony, and she ordered the murder of Ptolemy xv. It has been suggested that she was not a great beauty, but that her seduction of Mark Antony was accomplished by her lavish use of perfume. It is recorded that on one occasion she used unguents to the enormous value of 400 denarii just to soften and perfume her hands. She could afford to: at that time she was the owner of a 'balsam garden' which, by today's standards, was worth millions. After Antony's defeat by Octavian, and the death of Antony and Cleopatra, in 30 BC, Egypt became a Roman province.

The Romans were even more lavish in their use of perfume than the Greeks. Their perfumes were enclosed in bottles, *unguentaria*, usually of alabaster, onyx, or glass. Those for the bath were kept in a round, ivory box called a *narthecium*. The Roman perfumers, *unguentarii*, were numerous, and occupied a particular quarter of the town, the *vicus thuraricus* in the Velabrum. In Capua, a city noted for its luxury, they occupied a whole street. The Romans used three kinds of perfume, 'Ladysmata', solid unguents, *stymmata*, scented oils, and *diapasmata*, powdered perfumes. The names of solid unguents included *rhodium*, which was rose-scented, and *narcissum*, from narcussus flowers. Perhaps the most celebrated scented oils were *susinum*, which was made from honey, calamus, cinnamon, myrrh, and saffron, and *nardinum*, which included calamus, costus, cardamon, melissa, spikenard, and myrrh. Some of these preparations were very expensive, selling for as much as 400 denarii per pound. The Romans used them to scent their hair, their bodies, their clothes, their beds, even their military flags and the walls of their houses. Large amounts of scented oils and unguents were used to massage the body in the public baths, as well as at home.

Ovid, the poet of love, wrote a book on cosmetics, *Medicamina Faciei*, of which only a fragment has survived. He recommends frankincense as being an excellent cosmetic, saying that if it is agreeable to gods, it is no less useful to mortals. Mixed with nitre, fennel, myrrh, rose leaves and sal ammonica, he gives it as an excellent preparation for toilet purposes. Honey was the principal ingredient of all facial masks, and is included in another of Ovid's recipes, along with lupin seeds, beans, red nitre, and orris root: this was made up into a paste to removed blemishes from the skin.

The word 'anoint' means to rub, or to massage. Whether it was used in religious ceremony, healing, or simply to soothe aching muscles, aromatic massage has been in use for a long time. Certainly one of the greatest healers of ancient time was Jesus Christ. He also used aromatic oils in healing:

> 'On some he laid his hands, and they were healed; to others he just spoke the word, and they were full restored to health; but others had to go and wash in certain pools; and others he anointed with a holy oil' (The Aquarian Gospel 74. 3).

Just before the Last Supper Jesus himself was anointed, this time for a purely spiritual reason:

> 'Then took Mary a pound of ointment of spikenard, very costly, and anointed the feet of Jesus, and wiped his feet with her hair: and the house was filled with the odour of the ointment' (St John 12. 3).

Some of the disciples, with less understanding than Mary, actually rebuked her for using such an expensive ointment.

In *The Jesus Scroll* it is suggested that the 'Garden of Gethsemane' is a mistranslation, and that it was in fact known as the 'garden of Jessamine', the jasmine garden. The author also puts forward some very impressive evidence that the stone used to cover Jesus's tomb in the garden was actually a stone used in the making of jasmine oil. The flowers in the garden were picked, placed in a long, shallow trough of stone, along with olive oil, and then the stone was rolled along the trough. This pressed the essence out of the flowers, allowing the olive oil to absorb it. Whether true of this particular garden or not, this gives a very clear picture of a method for making scented oil, which was probably in use at the time. It is interesting to note that jasmine essence is today extracted by maceration in oil, because heat badly damages the quality of the essence.

When Rome fell the surviving Romans fled to Constantinople, and their knowledge of perfumery went with them. The splendour of Byzantium was a scented splendour. Trade in aromatic spices and gums became an important economic factor in the Holy Roman Empire. In spite of this the knowlege of distillation remained undiscovered or forgotten. It was an Arabian physician, 'Abu 'Ali al-Husain Ibn 'Abd Allah Ibn Sina, known in the West as Avicenna, who is credited with this 'invention' in the late tenth century. This extraordinary man found the time to write nearly one hundred books in a wandering life of fifty-eight years. At that time the Arabs had achieved great advances in matters of science, and the discovery of distillation was a natural result of their progress in the field of chemistry (or perhaps one should say alchemy). For his first experiments Avicenna chose one of the most cherished flowers of the East, the rose. He is said to have used the rose known as *'Gul sad bark', Rosa centifolia*. He also turned his attention to other plants, and distilled both essences and aromatic waters. Needless to say his discovery was soon put to practical use, and the fame of Arabian perfume spread. Rose water was one of the most popular scents and appears to have been manufactured in large quantities.[1] Rose water came to Europe at the time of the Crusades, along with other exotic perfumes and essences from the East. These products soon caught the eye of European businessmen, as well as the nose of the ladies, and by the end of the twelfth century Europe had its own manufacturing perfumers. In 1190 the French perfumers were granted a charter by Philip Augustus. At first many of the perfumes were copies of Eastern scents, but by the end of the thirteenth century Europe had started to establish its own fashions. Already lavender was being cultivated in Mitcham, Surrey, and lavender water was becoming popular.

The use of perfumes is not likely to have been overlooked by those ancient civilisations whose history is less well known to us. Minoan Crete and China both had civilisations even older than that of Egypt. Judging by their ancient knowledge of acupuncture one suspects that the Chinese may have used aromatics even before the Egyptians. The classic Indian herbal texts, the *Ayurvedas*, were written about the same time as the late Egyptian era. A great number of the preparations contain aromatics. Sandalwood has always been very widely used by the Indians, both in incense, beauty preparations, and in a holy unguent used to

---

1 Another, more romantic version of the discovery of rose essence is given in the chapter on the rose: see p. 274.

anoint the head of kings and high priests, as spikenard was used in ancient Israel (Judea). In India a cosmetic ointment known as *urgujja* is made, containing sandalwood, aloes, rose, and jasmine. Another ointment prepared with *usira* root (probably vetivert) was used to reduce fever.

Anointing the body with scented oil is still popular in parts of Africa, and helps to counteract the drying effect of a hot sun. They mostly use coconut oil or palm oil, scented with aromatic herbs or woods. Hutchinson, in his *Ten Years in Ethiopia*, speaking of a particular ointment called *tola pomatum*, says: 'The first thing of which one is sensible when approaching a village is the odour of tola pomatum, wafted by whatever little breeze may be able to find its way through the dense bushes.' The Arabs, copying a fashion initially used in ancient Egypt, make scented unguents in the shape of a cone. This is placed on the head and as it melts perfumes the whole body. Similar habits are practised in other countries with hot climates. In Tahiti the women wash their hair daily, and oil it with a pommade called *monoi*, made of coconut oil scented with sandalwood, or toromeo root.

A number of English manuscripts from the fourteenth and fifteenth centuries contain references to herbal oils, and instructions on how to make them. These are all infused oils, the aromatic herb being heated in oil. After a number of hours or days the oil is strained, and is ready for use. This is a method which was used by the Egyptians, and perhaps even before them. Surprisingly there seem to be quite a number of variations in the way these oils are made. The following extract is from an untitled work, the author of which is unknown. The manuscript, much of which is in Latin, contains several drawings showing different types of distilling apparatus. Though listed as *circa* fifteenth century, this particular part almost certainly dates from the fourteenth century. (In reproducing these manuscripts I have modified certain spelling conventions, and added occasional punctuation, to make the sense clearer.)

'To Make Oleum Mastycum.[1]

'Take a unce off Mastyke and a unce off whyte ffrankinsence or off alesander[2] made in pouder, and let them boyle well in a h[3] off oyle so styffe, and when

---

1 Mastic   2 Alexander, probably the name of a gum from Alexandria, perhaps a type of frankincense   3 Probably a hin

they have well boyled strayne it and kepe it tyll ye have nede to occupy[4] it.

'And iff ye wyll make it to help a mannys[5] stomake ffryst[6] take mynte . . . galingall[7] and boyle them well in ye oyle ffrust; and then putte yor other stuff and make up yor oyntment.

'And iff ye wyll have it ffor achs and payne off synowe[8] make yor oyntment off oyle rosary.[9]

'Thye oyle or oyntment off mastyke helpeth achie in the stomake and in the joynte in the shulders, raynys,[10] and other places [where] off it is a noynted a ffore and ffyer,[11] and it helpeth all dyssesys[12] off the lyver and the splene and ye must . . . and all warme kind if [applied] to your stomake or other place, ffor it is good ffor all colde causes.'

4 Use	9 Probably rosemary, or possibly
5 Man's	rose
6 First	10 Reins, i.e. kidneys
7 Galangal, an aromatic carmin-	11 Afore and after, i.e. in front and
ative root from China	behind
8 Sinews, i.e. muscles	12 Diseases

Mastic is a gum which is very similar to frankincense. Here we can see that the external use of aromatics for internal disorders is nothing new. Mint is included in the recipe for a stomachic oil, and frankincense for the liver, spleen, and various other parts. This oil is to be massaged into the body, both behind and in front of the affected part. If, for example, the stomach is being treated the oil is massaged into the upper abdomen, and into the back, at the same level. This front and back application of oil is now fairly standard practice in aromatherapy, and was probably being used long before the fourteenth century.

Many manuscript herbals contain similar recipes for oils, some of them also containing various unsavoury substances such as dried bees, flies, lizards, and even powdered roof tiles! Powdered 'tartar' was also a very popular ingredient. Here are some recipes from a manuscript entitled *An Herbal*, author unknown, which devotes a whole chapter to herbal oils.

'Here begynnyth the makynge of oyles of diverse herbys for dyvrse infirmytees, and first we shall describe the makying of oyle of laurel . . .

'Take berrys of laurell drye or grene and stampe

them small. And take an erthen pott with a lyd acordynge to this,[1] and put this in[2] a potell[3] of oyle or a galon, aftr the pott will receyve.[4] And caste this inne[5] that thu stampestest aforn,[6] and lyte[7] the lid and the pott wele togedr and sekterly, and sett it on the fyer on (top) of a tinete and this to make grete fyer. And lett it brene[8] fro[9] son rysynge to undern[10] or myddaye. And than clense[11] it throwe a clothe in to a fayr[12] vessell, and lete it kele,[13] and do[14] it in boxes and kepe it.'

1 i.e. which fits
2 i.e. 'in this'
3 A liquid measure equal to about half a gallon
4 'Depending on the size of the pot'
5 'In this'
6 Before
7 Seal
8 Burn
9 From
10 The third hour of the day; about 9 a.m.
11 Filter
12 Clean
13 'Let it cool'
14 Put

Oyle of Pulyoll ryall[1]

'Take the croppe[2] and the floures of pulyoll ryall and sette[3] hem in oyle in double vessell as it is aforesaid; and all evills of colde causes it dothe awey princypaly, and maketh a woman to conceyve.'

1 Pennyroyal
2 Tops
3 Steep

To Make Oyle of Herbys

'Take rewe[1] leves and stampe hem small, and lete hem rote[2] in oyle, vii dayes or viii, and sethe hem in double vessell as it is sayde in makynge of thy othr oyles.

'And this oyle is gade[3] for all maner colde causes, that is to daye for yliaca passis[4] and for the epylense[5] and for colica passis.[6]

'Wt[7] a noyntyng and wt aclisterye.[8]'.

1 Rue
2 Rot, i.e. mature
3 Good
4 Iliac pain
5 Epilepsy
6 Colic pain
7 With
8 Clyster, or enema

Oyle of Heye

'Take heye and lay it on the hote brennynge colys[1] and this of wyll reyse a smoke, and than take a plette[2] of yren and holde it a bove and the smoke wyll clene[3] this to and it will be sumdell[4] moyste; and what it is colde gadre it of and put it in a vyall of glas. And this oyle is gode for frekenes[5] and for the goute artatyk[6] and for the morfewe.'[7]

1 Hot, burning coals	5 Freckles
2 Plate	6 Arthritic
3 Cling	7 Morphew, a leprous or scurfy
4 Somewhat	eruption

This last method is a very simple form of distillation. Although distillation was known at this period, it was used primarily to make aromatic waters rather than essences. Aromatic oils were usually made by steeping the plant in hot oil. The *Grete Herbal* (sixteenth century) contains a very simple recipe for violet oil:

'Oyle of vyolettes is made thus. Sethe vyolettes in oyle and streyne it. It will be oyle of vyolettes.'

The earliest printed herbal is a book which has come to be known as *Banckes's Herbal*. The true authorship is uncertain, although it was probably a physician called Anthony Askham; but it was printed by Richard Banckes in 1527. It contains several recipes for rose oil:

'Oil of roses is made thus. Some boil roses in oil and keep it. Some do fill a vessel of glass with roses and oil, and they boil it in a cauldron full of water, and this oil is good. Some stamp fresh roses with oil, and they put it in a vessel of glass and set in the sun fifty days, and this oil is good against the chafing of the lives, if it be anointed therewith.'

Whatever method was used to make them, it is obvious that aromatic oils were widely used in the fourteenth, fifteenth, and sixteenth centuries. They were applied externally, but were made for a variety of internal disorders. They were probably made at home, as were aromatic waters, as well as by the local apothecary.

Thomas Norton, an alchemist from Bristol, was the author of a remarkable work entitled *Ordinall of Alkimy*, which was published in 1447. The following lines are extracts from his observations on odours:

'All things that is of good odor hath naturall heate though Camphir, Roses and things cold have sweet odors as authors have soules . . .
Also by odors this maie you learne,
Subtilness and groseness of matters to discerne.
A sweete-smelling thinge hath more puritie
and more of spirituall than stinking maie bee.
As colours changeth in your sight
So odours changeth the smelling by might.'

The herbalists and alchemists of the Middle Ages were as concerned with matters of heat and cold, or subtleness and grossness, as their modern counterparts are concerned with viruses and drugs. In an early thirteenth-century French manuscript we find: 'Olibanum est encens, il est chaud et seche el secunde de grei.' Every herb was classified in varying degrees of hot, cold, dry, and moist. Hot and dry qualities correspond to the Chinese yang characteristic, and cold and moist to the yin. There were four degrees of heat so a herb that was hot in the first degree was not quite as heating as a herb of the second degree. There were also four degrees of cold. This does not form an exact parallel with yin and yang. While the Chinese classified their remedies as yin or yang, European herbalists sometimes mixed a yin quality with a yang quality, so that a herb could be classifed as hot and moist, or cold and dry.

William Turner, commonly known as the father of English botany, was a sixteenth-century herbalist. He explains that herbs that are hot in the first degree 'increase the natural heat which cometh after the digestion and other natural workings'. those of the second degree 'are partaken of a fiery heat, therefore have no power to make subtle or fine, and to open the stoppings of the pores and other ways'. Those of the third degree, 'cut in pieces, they draw, they heat very much, and make a man thirsty'. And those that are of the fourth degree 'raise up bladders, burn and pull off the skin and fret inward'. As for essences, mustard oil would come into the fourth category.

Of the degrees of cold, he continues: 'Herbs and other medicines, that are cold in the first degree . . . cool the natural heat, and after some manner hinder digestion.' Those of the second degree 'make thick or gross, and evidently make dull, or minish the natural heat'. Those of the third degree 'Stop and shut up the inward ways and passages and the pores . . . make dull at the wits or senses'. And those of the fourth degree 'freeze together, or congeal, put out or quench the natural heat, and kill man if they take them in any great quantity'. This parallels almost exactly the Chinese concepts of yin and yang, and also relates to the four[1] elements: Air is hot and moist, Water is cold and moist, Fire is hot and dry, and Earth is cold and dry. The degrees and elements were also linked with the four humours: sanguine (Air), phlegmatic (Water), choleric (Fire), and melancholic (Earth). A predominance or lack of any one of the humours would indicate which element was too strong or too weak; this in turn would indicate which type of remedy to prescribe. This, in principle, is an exact parallel to the Chinese method of diagnosing and treating according to the state of the elements.

Another aspect of medieval herbalist was the doctrine of signatures. This was based on the idea that something about a herb — its shape, its colour, or some other quality — would indicate the part of the body or the particular disease which it would cure. This led to the naming of herbs such as lungwort, liverwort, and kidneywort, which vaguely resemble their respective organs, and which also happen to be beneficial for disorders of the same organs. Whether or not one feels that a herb resembles a certain organ is largely a subjective matter, and this kind of assumption is as easy to ridicule as it is to believe. Nevertheless there are some remarkable coincidences. The roots of couch grass bear a strong resemblance to the urinary passages and fallopian tubes, and are good for disorders of the same. Cypress nuts have a particular effect on the ovaries, which they strongly resemble. Plants with blue flowers, such as valerian and lavender, are sedative, and red plants, like cinnamon, cloves, and gum benzoin, are warming and stimulating. It is hardly surprising that the doctrine of signatures has been discarded, because one cannot generalise and say all plants with blue flowers must be sedatives. Roses, which have red flowers, are in fact sedative rather than stimulating, and so are camomiles, whose white petals surround an orange centre. Rose oil, however, is green, and camomile oil is blue: in fact the colours of essences give a more consistent guide than the colour of plants.

1 The Chinese in fact recognise five elements.

The influence of the planets must also not be forgotten. Nicholas Culpeper was the greatest, and also the last, of the astrologer-physicians. Though much respected during his lifetime, and ever since, for his knowledge of herbs, little respect has been shown for his astrological observations. I have little chance here to convert the disbeliever, and no need to preach to the converted; but the knowledge of astrology can be of great value in healing, and greater account should be taken of it than is done at present.

In addition to his great work on herbs, Culpeper published in 1660 a book entitled *Arts Master-Piece, or the beautifying part of Physick*. The introduction is headed 'To All Truly Vertuous Ladies' and includes the following:

> 'For these secrets of nature, by which nature has taught us how to beautifie, and make herself more comely, coming to my hands, I could not chuse but disperse them for benefit of those to whom I owe so great a respect . . . Therefore ladies, buy these few receipts, and make use of 'um, and if they fail, then never believe me another time; which displeasure of yours I would not willingly incur, out of my zeal always to appear, Ladies, your most faithful and devoted servant.'

The book consists entirely of recipes, some to colour the hair, some to colour the face, some for perfumes, and some for powders. There are also a number of recipes for ointments and oils for the hands, face, feet, hair, and so on. The great majority of these contain aromatic herbs, gums, oils, or waters. For example:

To make the breasts decrease or grow less

> 'The juice of hemlock mixt with camphure and layd on, makes them less; also white frankincense with navel-wort and sharp vinegar, hinders their growth.'

Another to make the hair grow again

> 'Take oyl of juniper, oyl of nuts, each one ounce, white honey, juice of dock each half an ounce, smallage seeds, asarabacca powdered, each two ounces, incorporate them and anoint the place.'

Another for the clefts of the hands

'Take of mastick, oyl of roses, white wax, each a
sufficient quantity, make an unguent.'

More recipes from this book are given in the section on 'Recipes'.
A great number of Culpeper's recipes contain rose oil, usually as
an anti-inflammatory agent. This, and most of the aromatic oils
mentioned, refer to an infused oil. A few essences are mentioned,
especially lavender; at that time they were coming to be used more
and more in 'physick'. As well as decoctions and infusions
Culpeper sometimes used oils to anoint the body in sickness.
Preventatives were also recommended, such as the following:

A Pomander for the time of Pestilence

'Take a labdanum, styrax-calmite, each one dram,
cloves half a dram, camphure, nard, nutmeg, each seven
granes, bruise them all to a fine pouder, and mix them
with rose-water in which tragacanth and gum-arabick
have been steeped, and make balls.'

The plague was the scourge of the Middle Ages, and during its
visitations fumigations were employed to destroy the supposed
'aura' or poison of the disease, which was generally believed to be
in the air. A seventeenth century medical writer recommends for
this purpose 'such things as exhale very subtle sulphurs, as the
spicey drugs and gums'. Among these he includes benzoin, styrax,
frankincense, and all aromatic roots and woods, and 'such drugs
as are from a vegetable production, and abound in subtle volatile
parts, [which] are of service to be exhaled into the air'.

During the Great Plague, fires were ordered to be lighted in the
streets at 8 p.m. and every twelve hours. Fires made with pine or
woods that gave out a pungent smell were thought to be most
effective. The Deanery of St Paul's was fumigated twice weekly
with sulphur, hops, pepper, and frankincense. Incense, in the
form of powdered gums, was frequently burned both indoors
and in the streets. Perfumed candles were burned in sickrooms
and hospitals; pomanders were hung from silver chains around
the neck, and perfumes were in great demand. Every aromatic
substance available seems to have been used in one form or
another to combat the Black Death. Aromatics were the best
antiseptics available at the time, and the people knew it. Exactly

how effective these measures were can only be surmised, but it has been widely reported that those in closest contact with aromatics, especially the perfumers, were virtually immune. Since all aromatics are antiseptic it is likely that some of those used were indeed effective protection against the plague. Up until the nineteenth century, medical practitioners still carried a little cassolette filled with aromatics on the top of their walking sticks. This acted as a personal antiseptic, and would be held up to the nose when visiting any contagious cases.

By the turn of the eighteenth century essential oils were being comprehensively used in medicine. Salmon's *Dispensatory*, of 1696, contains a recipe for an 'apoplectick balsam' including the oils of nutmeg, amber, roses, cinnamon, lavender, marjoram, ambergris, benjamin (benzoin), rue, cloves, citrons (lemons), civet, and musk.

> 'Mix all according to Art, to the just consistence of a Balsam. The oil of nutmegs is that made by expression, all the rest are chymical [essential] . . . It chears and conforts all the spirits, natural, vital, and animal, by anointing the extremities of the Nostrils and the Pulses. It cures Convulsions, Palsies, Numbness, and other Diseases proceeding of cold.'

The same book also contains a recipe for the loss of memory, using an amazing number of aromatics, which, summarised, include seven gums, three roots, eight herbs, three seeds, seven flowers, eight oils, and saffron. The instructions read: 'Pouder them that are to be poudered, them mix and distil in an Alembick, with a gradual fire; separate the Balsam from the Water', the 'balsam' here being a combination of essences. Whether such preparations actually cured conditions like amnesia or paralysis is doubtful.

The seventeenth century was the golden age of the English herbalists; Culpeper, Parkinson, and Gerarde were all of that period. Man's knowledge of medicinal herbs had grown considerably, but had not been overshadowed by chemistry. So popular had herbal medicine become that charlatans and quacks were quick to turn it to an advantage. As Eugene Rimmell writes:

> Itinerant vendors, or "charlatans", arrayed in a gorgeous red coat, with gilt lacings, addressed the gaping crowd from an elegant equipage, and dealt out

their perfumes and quack remedies with musical
accompaniment . . . they usually sold powders, elixirs,
pills, opiates, eau-de-Cologne, and scouring drops.'

Salmon's aromatic recipes are a curious mixture of genuine herbal medicine and quackery, and aptly reflect the then current state of affairs.

At this time, largely due to the appearance of such charlatans, herbal medicine began to lose much of its respect, especially among the medical profession, although they still used many herbs themselves. Joseph Miller's *Herbal*, written in 1722, contains references to a number of essences, thirteen of which are stated to be official preparations. These include camomile, cinnamon, fennel, juniper, bay, pennyroyal, rosemary, and thyme. Essences of juniper and thyme are the only official preparations of those plants. There are also four official infused oils: camomile, dill, myrrh, and rose, and one expressed oil, nutmeg

During the nineteenth century many essences were investigated more scientifically than had previously been possible. William Whitla's *Materia Medica*, first published in 1882, contains twenty-two official essences, and three unofficial. The official ones include camomile, cinnamon, juniper, lavender, lemon, peppermint, and rosemary. During the 160 years since Miller's *Herbal* was published, medical science had taken a great stride forward, and had long since left behind terms like 'heating' and 'drying' and 'opening obstructions'. Whitla's comments on myrrh include the following:

'Possesses the power, in common with other gum
resins, of stimulating mucous surfaces, and so influ-
encing their relaxed conditions in disease that the
abundant secretion is checked; thus bronchial catarrh
and chronic cystitis are improved; and it appears
likewise to relieve leucorrhoea and diminish secretion
from the cervical mucous surface.'

In the course of the scientific testing of the traditional uses of herbs at this time, their properties were sometimes upheld, and sometimes not borne out by the tests used. Most often herbs were abandoned in preference to chemical drugs, which acted more powerfully. However, essential oils were not seen in the same context as herbs, and, with the exception of a few herbal extracts have been more thoroughly tested over the last 150 years than herbs.

Although essences have had a chequered history in pharmacopoias all over the world for some time now, the general tendency has been to exclude rather than include them. Those that remain are, with a very few exceptions, only used as carminatives or flavouring agents. As well as diminishing in number, the pharmacopoeial oils have been credited with fewer therapeutic properties. This, however, does not reflect either the considerable therapeutic value of essences, or the degree to which they are used in medicine. In fact a considerable amount of research has been carried out since the turn of the century, especially with regard to the antiseptic properties of essences, vindicating their qualities and their usefulness.

This research has been principally conducted by chemists and pharmacists, and was initiated towards the end of the nineteenth century by Frenchmen like Cadéac and Meunier, and later doctors like Gatti and Cajola in Italy. In 1887 Chamberland published the results of his valuable research on the antiseptic powers of the vapours of many essential oils. During the nineteenth century the perfumery industry saw a steady, and considerable, growth. In those days perfumes were manufactured almost entirely from natural essences. As new oil-producing plants were sought, and land was found to cultivate them, the area around Grasse, in southern France, became, and still is, the world centre for the cultivation and extraction of essences. As the industry grew some of the companies at Grasse began to seek new applications for their essences; among these companies was the house of Gattefosseé.

René-Maurice Gattefossé was a chemist, and at first his interest (and his research) was confined to the cosmetic uses of essences. Two things happened which helped to extend this interest. Firstly cosmetics often contain antiseptics: Gattefossé had soon gathered enough information to convince him that many essential oils had even greater antiseptic properties than some of the antiseptic chemicals in use at that time. Secondly, one of Gattefossé's hands was badly burned when a small explosion occurred in his laboratory during an experiment. He instantly immersed it in neat lavender oil, and was only partly surprised when he found that the burn healed at a phenomenal rate, with no sign of infection, and leaving no scar.

Perhaps the first mention of the word 'aromatherapy', which was coined by Gattefossé, occurs in an article written by him:

> 'The French cosmetic chemists are concerned that the natural complexes should be utilised as complete building units in this instance without being broken up. Dermatological therapy would, thus, develop into "Aromatherapy", or a therapy employing aromatics in a sphere of research opening enormous vistas to those who have started exploring it.'

Here he echoes one of the basic tenets of natural therapeutics; that natural substances should be used in their whole, unadulterated form. This is an unusual viewpoint for a chemist, but he had found, from his experiments, that individual components of oils were not as effective as the whole essence: 'The whole is greater than the sum of its parts.'

In 1938 an article by Gattefossé was published which related the progress of a M. Godissart, a friend and colleague of his, who had recently set up an aromatherapy clinic in Los Angeles. He cites remarkable cures of skin cancer, gangrene, and osteomalacia, the successful healing of wounds which had refused to heal for years, facial ulcers which had been treated in record time, and 'bites from the Black Widow Spider until now considered to be fatal, are rendered harmless, thanks to the antitoxic power of lavender'. In fact the lavender oil combines chemically with the spider venom to form an innocuous compound. This also applies to snake and insect bites (and to other essences).

Gattefossé published his first book, *Aromathérapie*, in 1928. This was followed by a number of scientific papers and several other books, largely relating to therapy with essential oils. Although his work stimulated a great deal of interest this seems to have been largely dampened by the Second World War. For some 15 years after the war very little was published concerning aromatherapy, and research was at a low ebb. All was not lost, however: another Frenchman, this time a doctor, had been working for many years to re-establish the art.

Jean Valnet, a medical doctor, had always been interested in using herbs therapeutically when, no doubt inspired by

Gattefossé's work, he began to use essences in his treatments. During the war he used them extensively in treating battle wounds and soon realised, as Gattefossé had done, that here was a therapy with enormous potential. Since then Dr Valnet has used essences in the treatment of many pathological conditions, and is the author of many articles and a book, *Aromathérapie*, first published in 1964.[1] It is almost entirely due to his work that aromatherapy is now recognised as a therapy in its own right.

Italy has produced some notable researchers in the field of aromatherapy. The names of Drs Gatti and Cajola, who were working in the 1920s and 1930s, particularly deserve mention. Like Gattefossé they realised the enormous scope of therapy with essential oils, and their work ranges from the medicinal and psychological properties of oils to their use in skin care. Paolo Rovesti, director of the Instituto Derivati Vegetali in Milan, has produced many valuable contributions to aromatherapy in recent years. Most of his work has been with the citrus oils indigenous to Italy — bergamot, lemon and orange — and their deterpenated equivalents. He is probably the first person to demonstrate clinically the considerable benefit of certain essences in states of anxiety and depression.

About the same time as Dr Valnet was studying his essences Mme Maury, who died several years ago, was pursuing a similar, but even less orthodox, line of research. She was a biochemist, not a doctor, and did not feel confident about prescribing essences internally. Her interest was not strictly medical, and stretched into the cosmetic field. She searched for an external method of application which could serve both therapeutic and cosmetic purposes. This, of course, was nothing new; aromatics were being used externally, both cosmetically and therapeutically, long before they were ever used internally. But Mme Maury's work has been of great value. Continuing the more scientific approach of Gattefossé she formed the basis of a medico-cosmetic therapy based on massage, and made a thorough study of the way in which aromatics work physically, mentally, and cosmetically. In 1961, following the publication of several articles, she published a book, *Le Capital Jeunesse*, of which an English translation, *The Secret of Life and Youth*,

1 The English translation of this book is published by The C. W. Daniel Co. Ltd., Saffron Walden, Essex.

appeared in 1964, although at present our of print.[1] In 1962 she was awarded the Prix International d'Esthétique et Cosmétologie for her contribution to the field of natural skin care, and her book, largely based on her knowledge of ancient India, China, and Egypt, confirm this contribution and the message it contains. As an article commenting on the appearance of her book remarked:

> 'The French and Italian workers who are chiefly investigating this field of knowledge have at least more imagination than those who persist in regarding the human body as a more or less simple substitute for *in vitro* experiments.'

1 To be shortly revised by Danièle Ryman and republished by The C. W. Daniel Co. Ltd., Saffron Walden, Essex.

Chapter 3

Basic Principles

'The laws of nature are the laws of health, and he who lives according to these laws is never sick. He who obeys the laws, maintains an equilibrium in all parts, thus ensures true harmony; and harmony is health, while discord is disease.'

The Aquarian Gospel

Aromatherapy belongs to the realm of natural therapeutics. As such it is based on certain principles which are shared by acupuncture, herbal medicine, homoeopathy, etc. These principles are complementary, and are based on man's interpretation of nature from his understanding of life. To some extent this is bound to vary from person to person and from therapy to therapy. Nevertheless, there is an underlying truth towards which every school of thought is working. The closer we approach this truth the fewer contradictions there are, and the greater our understanding becomes. Surely the universe was created and is sustained on one set of principles, so there can only be one truth. If it were based on several contradictory ideas how could it possibly exist? It is only our individual interpretation of this truth which permits contradiction.

The main principles of our therapy are:

Life force

Yin-yang

Organic foods

45

Life Force

There is nothing more fundamental than life itself. It is the only thing we can be certain of sharing with every other human being. Whatever our spiritual beliefs or other differences, we are all alive. What is more we all believe in life; it is something we all take so much for granted that we hardly think of it as a belief although it is in fact a faith which we all share. Life in its essence is completely intangible; you cannot see it, touch it, smell it, or analyse it in any way. And yet we all believe that the sun will rise in the sky tomorrow, that flowers will bloom in spring, that we will continue to breathe for the next five minutes, and for the rest of our life, without any conscious effort. These things are manifestations of life. Life is present in everything. In a dried grain or stone or a dead tree, it is unmanifest, it has no movement, flow or apparent presence; it is there merely in form. But in a living thing — a plant or a human being — it is manifest, causing dynamic change, moving, flowing, loving.

The Chinese call it *Ch'i* (pronounced kee) the Indians call it *prana*, we call it energy, but everybody is referring to the same thing, the same life force that is keeping every one of us alive each minute of the day. There can only be one life force, one Truth, and that Truth is the only thing which we can be sure of having in common. If this life force exists (and who can deny it?) it must be the essence of everything — the force that holds the particles of an atom together, the power that makes a small seed grow into a tree, the attracting force of gravity or magnetism, the power that gives us consciousness. It is this same life force which manifests itself (in a slightly different way) in every plant. Just as we each have our own individual personality, so does each species of plant have its own personality or set of properties.

Extracting the essence of a plant is one of the ways of isolating this personality, but it is a delicate process. The life force is an extremely sensitive thing, and if we tamper with it too much it will lose much of its power. By careful extraction and storage the life force of an essence can be preserved, but the more an essence is interfered with, either chemically or physically, the more that energy, and its organic harmony, is reduced.

Fortunately most essences are extracted for their perfume, and the great care which is taken not to damage the scent during extraction also ensures preservation of the life force of the essence.

It is because essences are organic that they tend to work in harmony with the body. Very often they have a 'normalising' action. Garlic and hyssop oils, for instance, are good for both high and low blood pressure. Whatever the problem, they will tend to bring the body back to normal. This kind of effect is not seen in drug therapy; it is the prerogative of Mother Nature. This is why organic substances are comparatively harmless; they do not have the violent, calculated, impersonal action of drugs. Although they have certain properties, which they can be relied upon to produce, they also have an ability to adapt to the needs of different bodies and different people.

This same all-pervading life force is continually bringing about a state of health and harmony in the body. It is this power which is responsible for every activity taking place; it regulates temperature, blood pressure, respiration and the delicate balance of sodium, potassium, and all other chemicals in the body. When we break a bone all the surgeon can do is to set it; only nature can actually fuse the two broken ends together again. In fact we cannot heal the body, we can only encourage healing to take place.

The human body, like everything else, is in a constant state of activity and change. If there were not some central, governing, harmonising influence, almost every change that takes place would cause an imbalance resulting in disease. It is not our brain that performs this task. The central nervous system is merely one of the channels through which harmony is maintained. When you die your body is still intact, all its nerves are still there but something, which is not physical, is no longer present.

Our bodies are a miracle of divine engineering, which we could never hope to replicate; and they do not only contain flesh and bone, they contain us! So we are foolish if we treat our bodies as if they were overgrown test-tubes, filling them with chemicals, or as if they were cars, taking bits out when they go wrong. There are spare parts for a car, but not for this body.

If we recognise the existence of this life force, and that it is the only power which can produce health wtihin us, we will realise that we must work with it and not against it. We cannot heal directly; we can only help the body to heal itself by encouraging the natural healing force within, and allowing it to do what it wants to do. So often we interpret sickness as something unfortunate and undesirable, and yet often, especially in acute disease, it is a manifestation of the body's attempt to restore health and harmony.

Orthodox medical treatment very often suppresses the symptoms of disease, but if disease is in fact a healing process it should be encouraged. If you have filled your body with rubbish instead of food for years you may suddenly go down with influenza, gastroenteritis, or whatever. This type of acute attack is usually accompanied by diarrhoea and/or vomiting. Your body is trying to tell you that it does not want what you are eating, and is trying to get rid of some of the waste matter that has been building up inside it. When this happens you generally lose your appetite, and at this point a fast is usually indicated, and should be followed by a change in diet.

If we understand why the body reacts as it does, and what the real cause of the trouble is, then correct treatment can be applied. Chemical drugs tend to by-pass the natural healing force within the body, rather than working in harmony with it. Antibiotics are a prime example, killing off many harmless and useful bacteria as well as those which are harmful.

It may be that, hidden within every disease process, a healing process is at work, underlying the homoeopathic principle of 'like cures like'. In a minute dose a substance cures the kind of condition it would produce in a material dose. Essential oils can be used to suppress infection, in a similar way to antibiotics. It is not known exactly how they inhibit the growth of bacteria, but they do not have the unfortunate side-effects of antibiotics, because of their organic nature. Unlike chemical drugs they actually stimulate the natural healing force. This is demonstrated by the fact that a relatively small amount of essence, even applied externally, is able to rid the body of infection. In orthodox medical terms such a quantity would not be sufficient to dispose of the infection.

Yin and Yang

We use these two oriental words because we have no apt equivalent. Our nearest equivalent is positive and negative, or active and passive, but these have unfortunate connotations; we associate positive with good aspects, and negative with bad. Is day-time good and night-time bad? We often judge things as good or bad when really they are just one or other aspects of the same thing.

The physical universe was created when Oneness became duality, and we can see this duality, this yin and yang, everywhere in the universe, in every atom, every action, and in every function of the human body. Yin and yang are manifest everywhere, except at the very centre of being, the perfect point of balance, at that infinite moment when the future becomes the past.

In the very centre of a flower, a seed, or leaf bud, there is a point from which the energy is coming and from which growth proceeds. From that point the seed grows, the flower bud blooms. If you cut an apple or a cabbage in half you can see that it radiates from a central point. If you carefully examine the flower bud, leaf bud, seed, fruit, or vegetable, and dissect them until you come to their very centre, you will find . . . nothing. Really there is only one thing, one energy, one consciousness, but in order to manifest itself it becomes yin and yang. In striving for health and harmony we try to find that point of balance between yin and yang.

We can see yin and yang in the change of the seasons, the weather, the cycle of night and day. We can see it in the growth of plants; a seed needs earth (yang) and water (yin) to grow. From the shell of the seed a sprout bursts forth, and tiny roots begin to grow. The upward (yin) motion of the shoot is balanced by the downward (yang) motion of the roots. When the shoot bursts through the earth its environment changes completely. It is now under the influence of air (yin) and sunlight and heat (yang). The shoot (yin) develops leaves (outward: yang) and later flower-buds (yin), then flowers (yang) and fruit (yin). The fruit becomes more and more ripe (yin) until it finally falls to the earth (yang) and the cycle begins again.

Yin and yang can also be perceived at work within our own body. The circulation and respiration provide a perfect example. The heart contracts and dilates, the blood changes from red to blue and back again, and the breath goes in and out. Every single function of a living organism manifests these two forces. Obviously an understanding of their interrelationship and the way they manifest in the body, causing sickness or health, is an asset to any healing art. To know which oils are predominantly yin or yang gives a basic guide to their application in sickness.

Nothing is totally yin or totally yang; they are entirely relative terms. If we say that something is yin we mean that its qualities are more yin than yang. A herb or essential oil which is predominantly yang also contains yin properties. There is a constant transformation from one quality to the other. As the sun rises yin is diminishing and yang is increasing. When the sun reaches its zenith yang is predominant; at midnight yin is predominant. Both qualities are always present; there is no sudden change from one to the other.

Yin and yang always balance each other out, although they do not always neutralise each other. A storm is preceded and followed by calm. Hot weather makes the body lose more heat. A period of intense activity is followed by rest. Extreme hunger is satisfied by much eating! To every action there is an equal and opposite reaction. If sickness is caused by something yin the body tries to compensate by increasing one of its yang qualities, although this will not necessarily abolish the sickness. In some cases it may increase the yin—yang polarity, causing great stress.

Constipation is often interspersed with periods of diarrhoea. A fever is usually followed by a period of low activity with subnormal temperature. Lethargic depression is often interspersed by period of feverish activity, sometimes accompanied by elation: this is known as manic depression. A person may be very seriously ill, but not realise it because the increase of yin is counteracted by yang. Chronic disease is a state where there is a serious imbalance which has been artifically balanced: there are equal amounts of yin and yang, but they are not in the correct place in the body. The heart may be over-active and the kidneys under-active. The degrees of yin and yang may be balanced overall, but the body is still sick. In this case a remedy should be given which yinnises (sedates, cools) the heart and yangises (stimulates, heats) the kidneys. This will restore a true balance, bringing about a state of health. At the same time the reason for the initial imbalance may need to be treated, to prevent the condition recurring. This may lie in the body, the mind, or the environment of the patient.

Yin and yang are traditionally represented opposite:

This show yin within yang, and yang within yin, the one perfectly balancing the other. The 'S' shape in the centre represents the dynamic relationship between the two qualities. It also represents pure life energy — neither positive nor negative, but exactly at the centre of balance; not yang nor yin, and yet a part of both, because without that line neither shape would exist. It has no dimensions; it is infinitely thin and infinitely long, because it represents the wave of life energy that flows through everything. It is a two-dimensional representation of a spiral.

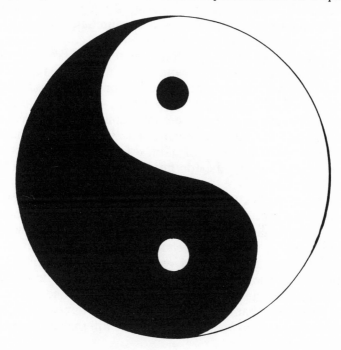

Organic Foods

'So eat always from the table of God: the fruits of the trees, the grain and grasses of the field, the milk of beasts, and the honey of bees. For everything beyond these is of Satan, and leads by the way of sins and of diseases unto death. But the foods which you eat from the abundant table of God give strength and youth to your body, and you will never see disease' (*The Gospel of Peace of Jesus Christ*, trs. E. Szekely and P. Weaver).

The importance of an organic diet in relation to health is at last becoming recognised by more and more people. Although there are several schools of thought — macrobiotics, vegetarianism, veganism — all agree on the importance of whole foods, as unrefined as possible and palatable. Being a vegetarian is more than just not eating fish and meat. In fact a new school of thought has emerged recently which advocates the eating of whole foods, including meat and fish, although unadulterated meat is not easy to come by. It is also, quite seriously, not very easy to eat a whole pig for lunch, let alone a cow for dinner.

Over-refined food (white flour, white sugar, etc.) is sadly lacking in life force, and this cannot be synthetically replaced in the form of added vitamins, minerals, or bran. Foods which contain artificial colourings, flavourings, or preservatives are slowly poisoning us. When we add vitamin C to blackcurrant juice we are disturbing the balance and harmony of a natural substance. The ingredients of natural foods are in perfect proportion to each other; they do not need to be added to or subtracted from.

The same applies to our medicines as our food. If they are natural, organic, and untreated they will work in harmony with the healing forces within us, helping that healing power to restore harmony to the body. Natural foods and medicines have been with us for thousands of years, unnatural ones only for a couple of centuries, yet already their usefulness and innocuousness is being seriously questioned. Scores of food additives and drugs have been banned because they are a danger to health. What about the ones we are using today, will they be banned in twenty years time?

Unnatural foods, by which I mean those which have been artificially processed in some way are a contributing factor to the general ill-health of the individual. In particular they tax the digestive and assimilative process of the body in such a way that these processes become inefficient. The results of impaired digestion and an unnatural diet are malnutrition and toxaemia. Over-indulgence of refined starch, as in white bread and cakes, may help to bring on a condition known as coeliac disease, in which wheat protein, especially in the form of refined flour, cannot be digested. Many adults as well as infants now suffer from coelic disease. The habitual eating of sugar, especially white sugar, may eventually lead to diabetes mellitus. This condition affects the ability of the body to control the metabolism of sugars.

The main function of the liver is to metabolise digested food. With the continual strain of having to deal with isolated chemicals, especially in the form of drugs, its efficiency may be impaired. This can lead not only to faulty metabolism but also to disturbances of the other functions of the liver. The result could be anaemia, which is due not only to faulty nutrition but also to faulty digestion and metabolism. Another consequence of the same problem could be cirrhosis, which is also associated with the excessive drinking of alcohol. Too many rich, fatty foods may lead to gall bladder troubles, and possibly gall stones.

There is now a government publication entitled *Diet and Coronary Heart Disease*, with over 350 references. The very fact that this study has been made is itself something of a landmark, and stands out against the general ignorance of the medical profession regarding dietary matters in relation to disease. Their ignorance is understandable, since diet is hardly touched on in medical schools. However, this ignorance has unfortunately given rise to a feeling among many doctors that diet and disease are completely unrelated, except for extreme nutritional deficiencies.

The DHSS report concludes that many factors contribute to ischaemic heart disease. One of these is obesity, which in turn is often caused by an excessive intake of sugar. Another is high blood pressure, which in some people can be lowered by a considerable reduction of common salt in the diet. The report also recognises that there is a definite correlation between the disease and the intake of fats, especially in the form of saturated fatty acids (basically animal fat as opposed to vegetable fat). It recommends that the consumption of dietary fat in the United Kingdom, which is steadily rising, should be reduced. It also recognises that an increase in the ratio of polyunsaturated (basically vegetable oils) to saturated fatty acids in the diet may cause a reduction in the amount of cholesterol in the blood. However, it clearly states that such a change in diet will not necessarily reduce one's chances of contracting ischaemic heart disease.

It is generally believed among natural therapists that excesses of sugar and animal fat in the diet are primary contributory factors to the incidence of heart disease, especially when the two are combined. It is believed that white sugar is more harmful than other, less refined, forms of sugar; hence the growing popularity of various types of brown sugar; and margarines and spreads, which are rich in polyunsaturated fatty acids. Sea salt is also believed to be less harmful than common salt. Of course these should also be eaten in moderation. Even if you are not in danger of contracting heart disease you can do no harm by keeping your blood pressure, body weight, and serum cholesterol content down to normal, healthy levels.

Another condition related to a defective diet is toxaemia. Toxaemia is a state of the body in which an abnormally high level of poisonous substances (toxins) is present in the tissues. These toxins are substances which are either not usually present in the system at all, or are kept down to a safe level by efficient elimination. General congestion of the system goes hand in hand with inefficient elimination. This state may be due to overeating, or simply faulty eating, and sometimes leads to obesity; it may, however, lead to other problems such as cellulitis or skin diseases. This state is something of a vicious circle. The eliminative organs cannot function properly if the whole system, including these organs, is being poisoned. The congestion, on the other hand, can only be relieved by elimination.

The toxins concerned come from two sources. Firstly they may be taken in with food in the form of artificial colourings, flavourings, preservatives, or chemical drugs, or they may be absorbed through the skin from cosmetics containing them. Many of these substances are only partially eliminated by the body, and in time they slowly accumulate in the tissues. Secondly, when a food such as white flour or white sugar has either been added to or devitalised, it is no longer in an organic form, and is often difficult to digest. In attempting to assimilate these 'foods' the body is actually robbed of some of its stored vitamins and minerals. Iron, for instance, cannot be digested without the presence of a trace quantity of copper. After they are digested these 'foods' often result in the production of toxins.

Some people feel no ill-effects from an unnatural diet, primarily because there are other factors at work which also influence the general state of health. Others will simply feel tired, listless, heavy, irritable, even though they may not have a definable disease. Others again will be affected more deeply, and may contract a skin disease: this problem is a result of the body's efforts to eliminate toxins which are in the blood, through the skin. Thus any treatment which suppresses this skin disease will only frustrate the body's attempt to heal itself, making the problem worse.

The most basic and simple treatment for this problem of toxic congestion is fasting. I need not elaborate on the history of fasting, but it is a very old therapy and, according to *The Gospel of Peace of Jesus Christ*, was practised by Jesus in healing the sick. The theory behind fasting is very simple. The body can safely go without food for anything between one and four weeks, depending on the state of the individual. Many people are under-nourished because their bodies cannot assimilate the inorganic food they are eating. It cannot do this because the assimilative mechanisms have been strained and partially damaged by long periods of bad eating. A fast will give the digestive organs a rest, and allow the natural healing power of the body to correct the faulty assimilative mechanism. In this sense fasting is sometimes able to cure malnutrition. A fast of longer than three days, however, should not be undertaken without proper medical supervision. By fasting I mean taking nothing except for water, which ideally should be pure spring water. Strictly speaking, if you eat anything else you are not fasting, although most people include a fruit juice diet under the heading of a fast. Grape juice is by far the best fruit juice to drink while fasting. It should be taken in wineglassful doses about every three hours; water may also be taken, as much as will satisfy the thirst. A fast should always be followed by a healthy, organic diet, otherwise the damage done by unnatural foods will simply return.

A healthy, organic diet is based on fruits, vegetables, grains, pulses, and a few high-protein foods. Fruits should consist mainly of fresh, and a little dried, fruit. Any vegetables in season may be eaten, either cooked or raw. Grains include rice, wheat, barley, oats, etc.; they should be eaten whole in the case of rice and barley, although wheat and oats are perhaps more palatable in other forms. Pulses include beans, peas, and lentils. Beans and peas may be either fresh or dried; there are many varieties of beans including soya, haricot, and kidney. Pulses are a very good source of protein, especially soya beans. Other high-protein foods include nuts, cheese, some seeds (e.g. sesame, sunflower), and yeast, which contains the highest percentage of vegetable protein, and is sold in many forms as yeast extract. Inevitably nobody will keep exactly to this diet; most will include such things as bread, butter, margarine, sugar, tea, coffee, and so on. The foods I have outlined form an ideal diet, and the closer we can keep to it the more healthy our diet will be.[1]

1 In the Therapeutic Index I sometimes refer to a 'non-toxic diet'. This is the kind of diet I am referring to. It is important to exclude alcohol, excessive quantities of tea or coffee, white bread, white sugar, and other over-refined foods, meat, fish, and poultry, and anything with quantities of chemical additives (flavouring, colourings, etc.)

I include a table of the protein contents of several foods, simply to demonstrate that it is not necessary to eat meat to ensure an adequate protein intake. Of course all the essential amino acids must be taken, but they do not all have to be taken in one food. The essential is for your diet to contain a variety of vegetable proteins.

Soya beans*	35.0[1]
Chicken (roast)	29.6
Peanuts (roasted)	28.1
Cheddar cheese	25.4
Sunflower seeds*	25.0
Roast lamb	25.0
Kidney beans*	24.0
Lentils (dry)	23.8
Haricot beans	21.4
Almonds	20.5
Cocoa powder	18.8
Pork chop (grilled)	18.6
Cottage cheese	15.3
Beef, average	14.8
Oatmeal	12.1
Eggs, fresh	11.9
Bacon, average	11.0
Brown rice*	8.0
Milk	3.3

1 All figures are in percentages, and are taken from the *Manual of Nutrition* published by the Ministry of Agriculture, Fisheries and Food, except those asterisked, which are taken from Frances Moore Lappe, *Diet for a Small Planet* (1971). Yeast is 52% protein.

Provided our diet is reasonably well balanced and organic, we need not worry about whether or not we are getting enough calcium, or vitamin B12, or any other nutrient. The amount of concern and anxiety that some people have about their diet is enough to triple their daily vitamin requirement in itself! If there is sickness in the body certain vitamins may be of benefit; these should be taken in the form of foods which are rich in those particular vitamins, rather than vitamin pills or capsules.

It has always amazed me how some people live quite healthily on hamburgers and coffee, while others seem to remain disease-prone, even on a diet of the healthiest foods. The fact is that our mental attitude generally, and particularly regarding our food, influences the relationship between diet and health. The more anxious we are the more vitamins we need, and the more likely we are to suffer from disease. A carefree, contented attitude is probably even more conducive to health than an organic diet.

The alchemists are remembered for their efforts to find the philosopher's stone, and to transmute one element into another in their search for gold. Lyall Watson suggests that the transmutation of metals was merely symbolic of the transformation of man into something more perfect. Colin Wilson describes this aspect of alchemy as 'man's attempt to learn to make contact, at will, with the source of power, meaning and purpose in the depths of the mind, to overcome the dualities and ambiguities of everyday consciousness'. The philosopher's stone was in fact a symbol of the key to this mystical knowledge.

The idea of transmuting elements was scoffed at by scientists until, in 1919, Ernest Rutherford proved that it could be done by bombarding elements with alpha particles. But all the time alchemists were searching for the key to transmutation, all the time scientists were scoffing at the idea and Rutherford, and others after him, were transmuting elements in the laboratory, transmutation was taking place inside their own bodies. It is happening now inside you, as you read. It has taken place in every plant and animal that has inhabited this planet. What was being so ardently looked for outside, was taking place within. In the same way the 'philosopher's stone', the key to spiritual knowledge, lies within us.

Louis Kervran is credited with the discovery that plants and animals transmute elements, although it was known to the ancient Chinese, who also knew that, in humans, it took place primarily in the liver. Kervran discovered that chickens can transmute potassium. Other experimenters have found that plants can thrive, producing a number of elements and compounds, from nothing but distilled water.[1]

If the transmutation of elements does take place in the human liver this explains why millions of people manage to survive on grossly inadequate diets, and I do not refer to the populations of 'underdeveloped' countries. On the other hand liver damage,

1 See Peter Tompkins and Christopher Bird, *The Secret Life of Plants* (1973) for further details of this phenomenon.

such as that caused by alcoholism, may lead to an impairment of the ability to transmute. Alcoholism is commonly associated with malnutrition, which is usually put down to lack of appetite. Whenever there is malnutrition, or a deficiency in the body, the health of the liver should be examined.

The principal known function of the liver is to metabolise digested food, breaking down certain substances and synthesising others. Included in its functions are: deamination of protein, desaturation of fats, synthesis of vitamin A, and formation of plasma proteins, albumin, globulin, prothrombin, fibrinogen, heparin, antibodies, and antitoxins. Because of its high level of activity the liver produces more heat than any other part of the body. If transmutation takes place anywhere in the body it must be in the liver, where there is such a high level of energy. Transmutation is a natural part of supplying the body with substances it needs, and this is primarily a liver function.

As long as it is being supplied with all the basic materials (proteins, carbohydrates, trace elements, etc.) the liver can probably manufacture any substance required by the body. However, if these materials are not in an organic form this will impair the liver's ability to metabolise in general, and to transmute in particular. We do not know how living things transmute elements, but we know that it is not identical to the process used by Rutherford, because this would be impossible. It must take place in a way peculiar to living organisms, and it is logical to assume that organic foods will lend themselves more readily to this process, and that unnatural foods may, in time, damage this function.

Even more important than the effect of unnatural foods is the effect of the mind. Anger, hate, frustration, jealousy, anxiety are all likely to cause liver damage, or at least hinder the liver's ability to metabolise and transmute. Any form of worry can cause physical sickness. In a recent report it is suggested that many severely neurotic patients tend to die prematurely without obvious physical illness, and that there is a much higher proportion of deaths among neurotics than would be expected.[1]

When treating nutritional deficiency, or simply poor nutrition, it is not always sufficient to recommend dietary supplements or a change in diet. Although this should certainly be done, it may also be necessary to treat the liver in particular,

1 See London *Evening News*, 5 March 1976.

and related emotional disturbance. For both of these purposes essential oils can often be of use. A short fast is usually beneficial in such cases, helping to clear the mind, as well as the body.

The fact that we can transmute elements under certain laboratory conditions does not explain how transmutation can take place in living organisms, where these high-energy conditions do not apply. The fact that we cannot understand it, although we know that it happens, is very frustrating, but it simply reflects on our real lack of knowledge regarding the nature of matter and of life itself. Perhaps we will find the answer by experimenting with plutonium reactors or cyclotrons; perhaps, on the other hand, we will find it in that mystical knowledge that the alchemists searched for so eagerly.

> 'This sovereign wisdom is so high
> That no reason nor science
> Can ever unto it attain.
> He who shall overcome himself
> By the Knowledge which knows nothing
> Will always rise,
> All thought transcending' (*St John of the Cross*).

Chapter 4

Odours

'If odours may worke satisfaction, they are so
soveraigne in plantes and so comfortable that no
confection of the apothecaries can equall their
excellent vertue.'

John Gerarde

Primitive man certainly used his nose more than we do today.
Even if we wanted to follow each other's tracks, by sniffing the
ground, what chance would we have of succeeding? Most of us
live in a highly polluted atmosphere, and eat a mucus-forming
diet; if you smoke you have even less of a sense of smell. Only
by fasting can you rediscover the acuity of your senses,
especially the sense of smell. You can then appreciate the depth,
beauty, and subtlety of, say, the odour of a fresh apple. It is
almost like a glimpse into another world: you realise how our
perception of the world is entirely dependent on the senses we
use to perceive it. Thus although we all live in the same world, in
a sense we live in entirely different worlds, according to our
perception and interpretation of things.

This is how important our senses are to us. Our nose is
probably less important to us than our eyes or ears, but it too
has its value. The sense of smell forms the greater part of what
we normally think of as our sense of taste. When you have a
cold, and your nose is blocked, your tongue can still taste quite
well, but the function of smell is impaired. Although we may
know, intellectually, what foods we like, and what a balanced
diet consists of, we still rely very much on our nose to guide us

in cooking and preparing food, and our enjoyment of food is primarily a nasal phenomenon.

Just as the ear distinguishes between noise and music, so the nose distinguishes 'bad' and 'good' odours. Bad odours are often associated with lack of hygiene, putrescence, and disease. In recent years, for example, air pollution has become a serious problem, but even coal smoke, car fumes, and industrial waste gases do not produce the stench that permeated the cities of Europe in the Middle Ages. When the dustmen go on strike for a few months we are reminded of what it used to mean to live in a city. Dan McKenzie comments on early nineteenth-century Edinburgh:

> 'And the whole stew was quite innocent of what we call drainage. Quite. Yet the waste-products of life, the lees and offscourings of humanity, all that house-maids called "slops", had to be got rid of. Very simple problem this, to our worthy Edinburgh forefathers. After dark the windows up in these "lands" were thrust open, and with a shrill cry of "Gardy-loo" (*Gardez l'eau*) the cascade of swipes and worse fell into the street below with a splash.'

Evil smells have always been counteracted by pleasant aromatics. If before the seventeenth-century the Englishman knew little of bathing, he at least knew, and used, plenty of perfume. The Egyptians mummified their dead with aromatic gums and spices; aromatics were used to counteract the plague, and holy or royal places and personages were always well incensed or perfumed. Each disease, too, is said to have its own individual smell. Dan McKenzie comments:

> 'Physicians of the last generation used to speak of typhus fever as having a close, mawkish odour, and the smell of smallpox is horrible. . . . There are others, however, less powerful and repugnant . . . the acid smell of acute rheumatism for one, and I have sometimes thought I could detact a characteristic odour also in acute nephritis, a smell resembling that of chaff. The odour of a big haemorrhage is unmistakable and, to obstetricians particularly, ominous.'

One might add that in diabetes the breath and urine usually smell of acetone, the smell of nail-varnish remover.

A sweet smell is said by Bacon to attend the plague:

> 'The plague is many times taken without a manifest sense, as hath been said. And they report that, where it is found, it hath the scent of a smell of a mellow apple; and (as some say) of May-flowers; and it is also received that smells of flowers that are mellow and luscious are ill for the plague, as white lilies, cowslips, and hyacynth.'

Here again we can see the homoeopathic principle of *similia similibus currentur*, like cures like.

The smell of the breath, perspiration, urine, and faeces present a subjective, but nevertheless practical aid to diagnosis — an unattractive guide but one much used by doctors of previous centuries.

Some of the most infectious diseases, have the most abominable odours. Is it not appropriate that the most pleasant and odoriferous healing agents are also the most antiseptic? They not only cover up bad smells, but effectively destroy the bacteria that cause them; hence their use as air fresheners, deodorants, and antiseptic agents.

Although man's sense of smell is not as acute as that of a dog or moth, we have, in theory, quite an acute sense of smell. As little of one part of ethyl mercaptan in two thousand million parts of water can be readily detected by the human nose, and distinguished from plain water. This is an exceptional example, a more representative figure being one part in 10,000. A slightly higher concentration, 1:1,000, is necessary to distinguish which odour is being perceived. Man also has the ability to distinguish between many thousands of different odours.

Surprising as it may seem we still do not know exactly how odour perception takes place; we have a much more thorough knowledge of sight and sound perception. This is not through lack of information regarding the structure of the olfactory sense organ, but its functioning is still something of a mystery. The roof of the internal nose is lined with a thin layer of mucus. Into this mucus project very tiny hairs; it is not certain whether the hairs project beyond the mucus, or simply into it. They form the tip of the rod-like olfactory nerve cells, and there are between six and twelve hairs to each cell. The hairs are unprotected extensions of the actual neural cells, so that olfaction is exceptional among the senses in that it involves an extremely direct interaction between the neuron and the source of stimulation. The other end of each neuron leads directly to the olfactory bulb in the brain. Olfactory stimulation, then, has the capacity to produce immediate and direct effect on the nervous system.

Air movement is necessary for continued olfaction to take place. This is because the odoriferous molecules 'use up' their energy in a very short period of time, and have to be replaced by fresh ones. Another attribute of odour perception is 'fading'. If the same odour is inhaled for more than a few seconds, the smell begins to fade, and may disappear entirely. This effect is more pronounced with some scents than others. Dan McKenzie observes that it hardly seems to take place at all when we are confronted with the most unpleasant odours!

The above facts demonstrate that the sense of smell is more dynamic than any other sense. Its effect is immediate, and then fades; it is not constant like the other senses. The fading effect can be counteracted by smelling a different odour, but there is also the effect of 'tiring'. Even if you keep smelling different things, after a while olfaction becomes less and less acute, until you can hardly smell any longer. Our bodies seem to be telling us that very little is quite sufficient when it comes to odours. Perfumers always work with dilutions of odorous materials, rarely, if ever, using them neat. Even so the effects of 'fading' and 'tiring' naturally present problems. They also have to cope with the fact that most odours have some effect on the body, in particular the nervous system.

Soap, Perfumery, and Cosmetics carried an article on this problem in July 1975:

> 'It must be remembered that ancient and recent investigations emphasise the pharmacodynamic activity of essential oils and their chemical components. In this respect they possess between them in varying degrees antiseptic, revulsive, hypnotic, aphrodisiac, tonic, vesicatory and analgesic properties. It would not therefore be surprising if among all these raw materials, both natural and synthetic, there are not some which are responsible for sensitising the organism, which take the form of attacks of illness following the inhalation of the vapours given off.

Phenomena of transient poisoning and local irritation
are manifestations of this.'

Headache, nausea, and allergy are also mentioned. The prolonged inhalation of any essential oil would eventually cause
headaches or other symptoms. The inhalation of many different
oils, one after the other, produces a faster and more pronounced
reaction.

It should be emphasised, however, that essences are powerful
therapeutic agents, and should always be used in moderation.
The inhalation of several different essences is bound to confuse
the nervous system, until, if you persist, it will produce violent
headaches and extreme nausea. This does not apply in the same
way to a blend of essences, that is to the simultaneous use of
several different oils. In this case their properties combine, or
balance each other, to form a product with its own individual
properties. A blend of oils does not have any worse effect than a
single oil.

Negroes reputedly make better perfumes than white men: their
perception of odours is thought to be more acute. This is connected with the fact that the olfactory cells, and the epithelial
cells surrounding them, are pigmented. This presents an obvious
parallel to the process of colour vision, which has been shown to
involve several pigments. The role of the olfactory pigment is
unknown, but we can speculate that it is as important to the dif-
ferentiation of odours as the ocular pigment is to differentiating
colours. In these pigments we can see a correlation between
odour and vision, which may be simply two different types of the
same vibration.

It seems likely that odours give off vibrations which fit into the
known electromagnetic scale. Daniel McKenzie postulates that
there may be two types of odour perception mechanism, which
operate simultaneously. One type is chemical, and depends on
odoriferous molecules being actually inhaled; the other type is
vibrational, and through this mechanism odours can be perceived
even if no molecules reach the nose. He cites the case of a female
Great Peacock moth, which attracted dozens of males from
several miles distant, even though they were flying against the
wind, and so her scent could not have reached them.

This type of theory is not to be confused with modern vibrational theories of odour perception, which postulate that

odoriferous molecules, which vibrate at different frequencies in different substances, communicate their vibration to the olfactory hairs. This theory is becoming very popular — and also controversial since it has its opponents. R. H. Wright, an American researcher, published a paper in 1954 stating that, if odour perception is associated with molecular vibration, the frequencies involved must, on quantum and thermodynamic grounds, correspond to the infra-red part of the spectrum. Here again we can see a correlation between colour and odour. Infra-red rays are so close to the visible spectrum that we can call them 'invisible colour'. What are scents if not invisible colours? In Krippner and Rubin's *The Kirlian Aura* it is suggested that if the sense of smell is connected with electromagnetic waves, one might expect the skin to be senstivie to odours. This is not as far-fetched as it may sound. We know that the skin is especially responsive to essential oils, but much more impressive is the fact that some people can see with their skin. In Russia ordinary people have been trained to distinguish colours by touch, after only a few hours' tuition. Each colour is said to have its own texture; yellow is 'slippery', red is 'sticky'. They have also learned to distinguish colours without actually touching the object. Rosa Kuleshova, who was very thoroughly examined by the Soviet Academy of Science, can actually see with her hands and elbows, and read newsprint without even touching it. If people can see with their skin, perhaps dermal odour perception is possible.

Under the influence of hallucinogenic drugs such as LSD the senses often become confused. One can 'hear' tastes, 'smell' colours, and 'see' music. Obviously there is some correlation between colour, odour, and sound. All three have a healing potential which could possibly be combined. It is a subject worthy of further investigation. Another modern theory of odour perception relates to the shape of odoriferous molecules. J. E. Amoore has demonstrated that round molecules smell camphoraceous, disc-shaped molecules have a floral odour, and wedges smell similar to peppermint. This does not contradict the vibrational theory, and they may eventually prove to be two aspects of the same phenomenon. Shape is also a product of vibration, as well as odour, colour, and sound.

McKenzie's theory of a 'subtle vibration' rather than a physical vibration has more to do with the sixth sense, with extra-sensory perception. Every object has a subtle vibration, which produces and dictates its shape, odour, colour, or sound. A sensitive person can detect this vibration directly, without the need of external senses. In this way a healer picks up the vibration of disease. He may be able to tell from its vibration, not only where it is, but also what it is. He may use his own body to produce a healing vibration, or he may use a healing agent, such as an essential oil.

Essential oils are natural, organic substances. They are like milk in a mother's breast — a part of the plant, and yet a separate substance from the rest of the plant. As long as they are kept in proper conditions after distillation they will not lose their organic quality and hence their therapeutic value. Although the properties of essences are not always exactly the same as the plants they come from, essences do 'represent' herbs to a large degree. The essence may not contain all the chemical constituents of the herb, but its vibration is similar, and it usually turns out to have the same properties. The essence is not the herb, but speaks for the herb, and has the same personality. The essence, as its name implies, is more concentrated and subtle than the herb; it acts on higher levels, and has a more pronounced emotional effect.

Why natural oils? Why not anything that smells nice whether it is natural or synthetic? The answer is simply that synthetic, or inorganic substances do not contain any 'life force'; they are not dynamic. Organic substances are those which are found in nature, like essential oils. 'Organic' also means 'structural' something which is 'characterised by systematic co-ordination of parts in one whole'. Nature has a structure which cannot be duplicated artificially. We can synthesise chemicals, but we cannot structure them to make something organic. Take an apple, and put it through a juice extractor. You get juice out of one end and pulp out of the other. Now put the apple and the pulp back together again. Do you get an apple? The structure of the apple is destroyed, and no scientist in this world can duplicate that structure. We now know from experiments in Russia with Kirlian photography that every living, organic substance gives off radiations, which can be seen as light. This is a manifestation of 'life force', the power which gives life. We also know that inorganic substances such as drugs usually have unfortunate side-effects which are often cumulative, and may not become apparent for some years. Everything is made of chemicals, but organic substances like essential oils have a structure which only Mother Nature can put together. They have a life force, an additional impulse, which can only be found in living things. It seems logical to suggest that the comparative harmlessness of organic substances has something to do with the fact that they are natural; that a man and a flower are both being sustained by the same life force, and are therefore in harmony; that the organic structure of the flower renders it comparatively harmless to the organic body of the man; that the beneficial effect obtained from herbs such as the Bach flower remedies is as much due to their life force (and their organic structure) as it is to their chemical constituents.

Although the composition of most essential oils is complex it is now possible to make a complete analysis of their chemical constituents. The oil can then be artifically reconstituted by combining the same chemicals in the correct proportions. The only reason for following this process is that it can prove cheaper than using the natural oil. The odour of reconstituted oils is never superior to that of natural oils; the reverse is usually the case. Neither, as one would expect, can they compare with natural oils as far as therapeutic potency is concerned.

The tools of aromatherapy are natural, botanical essences and vegetable oils. We never use aromatics from animal sources such as civet, musk, and castoreum. Not only do these substances come from the intestines or sex glands of animals, but they necessitate the death or suffering of the animals involved. The vibrations of death and suffering have no place in healing. For the same reason we do not use fatty oils such as turtle, spermaceti (whale-oil), and fish-liver oil. Needless to say, this goes hand in hand with the vegetarian principles of natural therapeutics. Neither do we use mineral oils, for these come from dead, inorganic sources with no natural life force, and therefore can be of no real therapeutic value.

Modern research and analytical techniques have enabled us to establish, in many cases, why a particular herb is good for a particular condition. This has reinforced much of the ancient empirical knowledge. We now know, for instance, that the essential oil from camomile flowers contains a substance called azulene. Azulene (so called because of its blue colour) is an anti-inflammatory agent, hence the effectiveness of camomile in cases of itching or inflamed skin, conjunctivitis, etc. (Incidentally it is interesting that azulene should be blue, since blue is at the opposite end of the spectrum to red, the colour of inflammation.)

Azulene is often used (in isolation) in skin creams. However, just because a certain constituent is largely responsible for the action of a herb does not necessarily mean that this 'active ingredient' will be more effective if it is isolated or synthesised. In Dr Valnet's book *Aromathérapie* we find this passage (my translation).

> 'The natural, unadulterated essence has proved to be more active than its principal constituent. . . . In 1904 Cuthbert Hall demonstrated that the antiseptic properties of eucalyptus oil are much greater than those of its main constituent, eucalyptol.'

It may be that the reason for this is that the minor constituents have a synergistic (controlling) effect on the main one. We come back to the idea of an organic, structured whole, which, if it is broken down, will lose some of its beneficial effects. Kirlian photography has shown us that the aura of a leaf fades as the leaf dies. In the same way the life force, or aura, of an organic substance is broken down when that substance is broken down.

We have already seen that the external use of scented oils and waters for internal disorders has a long history. Probably the earliest form of aromatic therapy was smoking or fumigation. This was practised in ancient Egypt and Babylon, and in Anglo-Saxon England. Originally the practice of smoking was hardly distinguishable from that of burning incense. It was used primarily in nervous disorders, to cast out evil spirits, and as a process of purification. Women often underwent fumigation during the menstrual and puerperal periods. This may have been because they were regarded, at those times, as being unclean; it may also have been that the herbs used had a beneficial effect in the circumstances.

Theophrastus spoke of the medicinal properties of perfumes, and of the effect of plasters and poultices on tumours and abcesses. He wrote: 'If one lays a plaster on his abdomen and breast, he produces fragrant odours in his breath.' English herbalists of the fourteenth and fifteenth centuries often used anointing oils in the treatment of sickness. This extract is from one of the oils mentioned in *An Herbal*:

'And if a man by a noyntid this wt fro the navle donne
to the pvyte be hynde and be fore it dothe a wey the
ache oute of the veynes. And if a woman by a noyntid
this wt in the same manr it clenseth the matte and
make hir able to conceyve.'

'Pvyte' refers to private parts, or genitals; 'matte' may refer to
matrix, or womb. The oil concerned is difficult to decipher, but it
looks like 'junipe'. Massaging the oil both behind and in front of
the affected part is a most effective method of external treatment
with aromatic oils.

Herbs are also used externally in the form of decoctions and
infusions, which are applied either as baths or compresses. The
most renowned exponent of this type of herbal medicine is a
Frenchman, Maurice Mésségué, who recently published an auto-
biography entitled *Of Men and Plants*. Mésségué always uses his
herbs externally, and always picks and dries his own herbs. His
treatments have been so effective that, from a simple village pea-
sant, he became a healer of great standing, treating men like
Winston Churchill, Konrad Adenauer, and Prince Ali Khan.

After many years' practice as a herbalists he is able to look
back on a considerable degree of success. One of his colleagues
compiled a list of ailments which he had often treated. The
percentage figures for completely cured cases include 98% for
eczema, 80% for insomnia and migraine, 60% for asthma, and
30% for chronic rheumatism. How much of Mésségué's success
is due to his herbs, and how much is due to the man himself is a
matter on which we can only speculate. His knowledge of herbs
was largely passed on to him by his father, who had probably
learned from his own father.

Mésségué only uses a small selection of herbs, about half of
which are aromatic. These include camomile, lavender, melissa,
mint, rose, sage, and thyme. Treatments are only applied externally, and include foot and hand baths, hip baths, vaginal
douches, poultices, compresses, and gargles. These treatments
are primarily used at home by the patient, and are usually
employed at least once daily. The history of aromatic waters is as
ancient as that of aromatic oils, and runs parallel with it. After
the invention of distillation, waters were even more commonly
used in treatments than oils, and most homes had their own
'stills'. The more wealthy households had a special room for

distilling fragrant waters, and this duty was performed by the 'still-room maid.'

We can reconstitute aromatic waters by mixing essential oils in water. The result is not exactly the same as a distilled aromatic water, but the two have similar properties and vibrations. Aromatic waters are excellent products for all the applications mentioned above. Further details of their uses are given in the chapter on baths. Although essences do not, strictly speaking, dissolve in water, a mixture of the two gives a product of excellent therapeutic quality, which lends itself to a number of different methods of application. Water is probably the best medium for absorbing vibrations and is, of course, basic to all forms of life. It seems to have a catalytic effect on essences, drawing out their healing force, at the same time having a tempering effect. It is as if the original balance of qualities in the living plant were being reconstituted, and yet the aromatic water is more subtle and dynamic than the plant itself.

Mességué's basic treatment consists of foot and hand baths. Exactly how these work is difficult to say, but the fact that they do work is incontestable, and they are more effective than ordinary, whole-body baths. It is interesting to note that the most important and most widely used acupuncture points are all below the elbow and below the knee.

Mme Maury does not appear to have used aromatic waters very much. Having searched around for the ideal method of external application she decided on a mixture of essential and vegetable oils. The skin has an affinity for oils, and vegetable oils are absorbed more readily than mineral ones. She saw that by massaging the body with aromatic oils one could combine the properties of the essences with the beneficial effects of massage itself. She also formulated the idea of an individual prescription: a mixture of four or five essences which were not only suited to the sickness, but also to the person. She realised that sickness is not an isolated incident, but is intimately related to the lifestyle, attitudes, and personality of each individual. Since no two people were exactly alike, everybody would require individual treatment. Like the homoeopath she would often alter the individual prescription as the patient's condition changed and improved. She rarely, if ever, used the same prescription on two different people.

Originally Mme Maury gave her clients essences to inhale. This proved to be a temporary and unsatisfactory form of treatment.

She was, in any case, dealing primarily with problems which affected the appearance: skin problems, obesity, loss of hair, and so on. She was not happy about giving essences internally, but she realised that they could also penetrate the body through the skin. She writes:

> 'If we could make the odoriferous matter penetrate directly through the skin into the extra-cellular spaces, and thus into the organic liquids in which the cells bathe; if we could diffuse this fluid matter within a reasonable time and at a reasonable rhythm it would be possible to establish a new treatment and find a new way. This at least would be safe, effective, and entail no risk.'

The cutaneous penetration of essences is slower, more diffuse, and therefore safer than inhaling or ingesting them. This kind of penetration takes place whether the essences are dissolved in oil or water. In the case of aromatic waters it may be only the odoriferous molecules which actually penetrate the skin, which is basically waterproof.

In order that effective dermal penetration can take place the skin itself should be in a reasonable state of health. If skin and body fluids are in a state of toxic congestion fasting or dieting should be undertaken in conjunction with aromatherapy treatment. Mme Maury made a thorough study of the cutaneous penetration of substances, with particular regard to essential oils. Her researches revealed that a substance which is introduced through the skin can actually diffuse through the body. She explains:

> 'This diffusion takes place by exchanges between the extra-cellular and lacunary[1] liquids and the blood, the lymph and the tissues. The elements introduced are carried by the liquids to the organs and retained selectively by the latter. This operation takes from three to six hours in a healthy individual and from six to twelve hours in the case of a thick congestioned body. Later, our own experience taught us that this time is considerably shorter in the case of a more transparent and diaphanous nature.'

1 The lacunary liquids are contained between pleura and the lung, the peritoneum, and all the other cavities.

When essences are introduced to the body through the skin they travel through the body fluids rather as hormones are carried in the blood stream, except that they are not limited to a particular fluid system, such as the blood. This method of application may be more effective than taking oils orally, in the sense that an adequate, steady diffusion through the body is assured. When an aromatic oil or compress is applied over an affected area the essences penetrate directly to the organ concerned.

Mme Maury found that her individual prescriptions often reflected the state of the client, rather than being an opposite vibration. This obviously relates to the homoeopathic principle of like curing like. By the time a 1% dilution of essence penetrates the skin and is diffused in the body fluids, the effect on the tissues must be something akin to a homoeopathic one. Aromatherapy is not actually homoeopathic but, when the essences are used in very small amounts, is more like applying the vibration of a plant than the plant in its gross form, or a set of chemical constituents.

Essential oils have varying rates of evaporation. The fastest, lightest oils are eucalyptus and orange, and the slowest and heaviest are patchouli and sandalwood. Between these extremes all other essences evaporate with varying velocities. This information is used by the perfumer to ensure a lasting and balanced product. He divides the evaporation scale into three sections: top notes, which are the lightest oils, middle notes and base notes. The base notes are used as fixatives, to 'hold back' the faster notes, and to make the scent last as long as possible. The top notes are the scents most noticeable when you first smell a perfume. The aromatherapist should also have a balanced product when mixing essences; not only for the sake of its perfume, but so that all of the elements are represented.

These three classes of essence also have their own characteristics. Mme Maury comments that base notes 'apply in general to the purely vegetable and cellular domain, and that the quality of the tissues is influenced'. One might add that base notes tend towards solidity and sedation, and should predominate in the treatment of those who are nervous, erratic, or flighty. Most of the gums and woods are included here; they act on the mucus membranes, and are valuable in chronic conditions. They were the earliest aromatics to be used, and may be useful in conditions of long standing, or which hark back to a childhood cause. They are often used for treating elderly people.

Middle notes primarily affect the digestion, the functions of the body, and the metabolism. They include most of the spices — cardamom, pepper etc. — and many of the herbs including lavender and peppermint. Here we also find basil, used to treat inability to concentrate or to digest information, hyssop for high or low blood pressure, and clary sage for menstrual malfunctions. At least one middle note should be present in all compositions to ensure that there is a link between the fast and slow elements, between the air and the earth.

The top notes are the fastest-acting essences, and should predominate where there is extreme lethargy, melancholy, or lack of interest. They are stimulating and uplifting, and include rosemary, juniper, and sage. These observations are intended as a general guide to help with the formulating of individual prescriptions: they should not be taken to cover every case. Just as we all have our own characteristic smell it is possible to formulate a blend of essences especially suited to each individual. Their physical and mental health should be taken into account, and also their personality, and attitude to life and to their sickness. Our health cannot be separated from the life we lead, and everything that influences that life.

Chapter 5

The Body

'That which produces harmony in all the parts
of man is medicine, ensuring health . . .

'The body is a harpsichord, and when its
strings are too relaxed, or too tense, the instru-
ment is out of tune, the man is sick . . .

'Now, everything in nature has been made to
meet the wants of man; so everything is found in
medical arcanes . . .

'And when the harpsichord of man is out of
tune the vast expanse of nature may be searched
for the remedy; there is a cure for every ailment
of the flesh.'

The Aquarian Gospel

A great number of aromatic gums, herbs, and their respective
essential oils came into medical use during the eighteenth century. As the nineteenth century progressed, and turned into the
twentieth century, a slow but sure trend was established. The
perfumery trade expanded, and at the same time pharmaceutical
research became more and more chemically orientated. The
discovery and synthesis of drugs became its central concern. The
earlier herbalists, who were more concerned with matters such
as humours, degrees of heat, cold, moistness, and dryness, and
so on, had succeeded in curing their patients, even without
knowledge of these drugs and their companion diseases. They
did not set out merely to suppress infection, but to make their
patients as healthy as possible — a more positive approach.

Sometimes the old herbalists used aromatics containing

essences which operated to suppress the infection anyway, but because of their ignorance of dosages, etc. their treatments were sometimes unsuccessful. By using the right combination of essences for each particular case or condition, however, we can improve on the success rate of the old herbalists, and at the same time do a great deal less damage, and more for the general health of our patients, than those who only use chemical drugs. Of course essences cannot do everything, and sometimes surgery, or antibiotics, need to be employed. But the world of aromatics contains a wealth of antiseptic agents, in the form of essential oils, about which so much research has been done that it is impossible to incorporate more than a fragment of the existing knowledge in this book.

The pharmacist will sometimes insist that he knows all about essences and their properties, but that in virtually every case he has found something more effective, more powerful, less expensive, and more synthetic. He might not tell you that the more powerful an agent is for good the more potentially harmful it is. Neither will he have much idea about the benefits of organic substances as opposed to inorganic ones.

The nineteenth century saw the gradual replacement of natural by unnatural medicines, while the perfumery trade took over the use of most of the aromatics. However, if you are to heal people, and not just contain disease, you have to be able to see further than the length of a microscope. For instance, take the case of the common cold. No drug as yet has been found for this complaint; indeed it will be a pity if one ever is, for it will be suppressing a natural process. Quite a number of American dollars have been spent in research to find the right drug to kill the cold bug. So far those erudite Yankee brains have failed to come up with anything, mainly because they have found that there are at least 113 different cold bugs! They cannot see what the physician of ancient times, with his doctrine of humours, could not fail to miss; that the treatment for a cold is heat. Not any old heat, but heat in the form of a natural remedy — black pepper oil, or clove oil for instance. On the other hand when the body becomes overheated, which is what we call a fever, one should give a remedy which has a cooling effect; oil of eucalyptus for instance.

If we are treating a disease which is associated with a bug, our choice of essences should not only be limited to those which neutralise that particular bug. Tuberculosis is associated with a bacterium. There are a few essences which are moderately effective against this bug, but we should also consider oils such as myrrh, which counteract the general state which TB produces in the body. The simplest way to explain this is in terms of the elements. TB is a cold, moist, watery complaint, and myrrh is a hot, dry, fiery essence. See the section on myrrh oil for a further explanation of its action.

I do not suggest that we ignore bugs but that, whenever possible, we use essences instead of chemical drugs, and that we understand that treatment should not be totally bug-orientated. It has often been suggested that bugs only attack us when we are in a very low state of health — when our resistance is low. When we are healthy and fit we are far less susceptible to infection. It has also been suggested that harmless bacteria, which normally live in our bodies, actually change into harmful bacteria when the chemical balance of their environment (i.e. the body fluids) becomes unbalanced. It is maintained that such an imbalance takes place in association with ill physical or mental health. Which causes which is a moot point, but if we remain healthy the bacteria remain harmless. Perhaps more virulent bugs can attack even the most healthy of us. Whatever the truth is, let us not get too obsessed with bugs. Ill health is more than just having caught a bug, and so treatment must take into account these additional factors.

Drugs, or essences, may be effective in suppressing infection, but the human body has the ability to fight them without any assistance or interference from outside. If it did not have this ability the human race would have died out many thousands of years ago. If you have influenza, and your doctor gives you an antibiotic, all he is doing is perhaps speeding your recovery by a day or two; you do not really need that antibiotic. And there is a growing and real problem with antibiotics. Because of their indiscriminate use, bacteria are becoming resistance to them. New strains appear, and new drugs have to be manufactured. It is a race which, once we have entered it, we can never quit, and it has no forseeable end.

I am not suggesting that essences should be substituted for antibiotics, although this may be a step in the right direction. Any substance which is powerful enough to be effective against a number of different conditions in millions of different people is bound to cause problems. The solution lies, rather, in reducing our dependence on them and paying greater attention to the positive health of the individual. When prescribed individually essences are almost as effective as, and far less dangerous than, synthetic drugs. But they should not be used solely for their antibiotic properties, or we will merely have a repetition of the same problems. A more individual and subtle approach to the treatment of ill-health is required — something akin to the homoeopathic approach — which will give the whole person the support they need in the right place, in the right way for them, so that harmony is restored and ill-health can no longer exist. In this sense essential oils can play a useful role.

Why is it that one person may contract cancer, or pneumonia, and live, and another may die from a cold or a bee sting? This is a question which is brought to the attention of the medical profession almost every day, as patients live or die in their hospitals. Two patients may receive the same treatment for the same condition, and yet one lives, and the other dies. There must be a difference between the two, and since it is not in the disease or its treatment it must be in the patients themselves. Our personalities, our attitudes, and our bodies are so varied, it is surely not surprising to expect that we need individual treatment when we are sick.

When prescribing essential oils we must consider all the present symptoms and other factors, whether psychological or physical. For instance, under 'bronchitis' you will find 14 different oils given. In order to ascertain which oil or oils to use you will need to know whether the condition of chronic or acute, whether there is excessive catarrh or not, whether the person is anxious or depressed, whether any other conditions (perhaps constipation or arthritis) are present, and so on. There is an essence — or blend of essences to match every disease pattern. Our task is to find the correct one.

Dr Valnet has commented that essences are often more powerful when given in greater dilution, but without actually being given in homoeopathic doses; by this he means without being diluted to an infinitesimally small concentration. In fact some essences, such as eucalyptus and sandalwood, are used in homoeopathic practice, and they are used in material, rather than infinitesimal, amounts (Boericke suggests eucalyptus oil in five-drop doses). Some aromatics, such as camphor, are used in the form of tinctures, which also contain a 'material' amount of essential oil. This, perhaps, is not true homoeopathy, which is principally concerned with potencies, but we can see how botanical and homoeopathic practice may overlap.

The prescribed dose of a given substance is a very important factor, in orthodox medicine, in homoeopathy, and also in aromatherapy. If given in the wrong dose, a substance will not produce the desired therapeutic effect, and may even do harm; sometimes it will actually have the opposite effect. Oils of melissa and rosemary, for instance, are either stimulant or sedative in action, according to the dose given. A high homoeopathic potency often has the opposite effect to a material dose; indeed this is one of the principles upon which the practice of homoeopathy is based.

Some homoeopathic medicines consist of poisonous substances such as arsenic or lead, but these are only given in potentised doses. Such essences, like mustard and wintergreen, are hardly ever given internally because of their high toxicity. They could, however, be given in very small doses. Essences are demonstrated to have certain therapeutic effects in certain doses. We normally assume that these effects will not take place if insufficient oil is used, but the practice of homoeopathic medicine shows us that any therapeutic agent, whether animal, vegetable, or mineral, continues to act on the body when given in smaller and smaller doses, although the nature of its action may change.

As regards giving essences homoeopathically, this is a subject which needs to be researched far more thoroughly before one can be sure of the action of a given oil, in a given potency. However, a potentised remedy is not just one which has been diluted to a certain degree, it is a little more complex than that. Not having been proven homoeopathically, therefore, essences must be given in small rather than potentised doses. Although, in the section on Essences, you will find a recommended therapeutic dose given for each essence there is nothing to stop you giving less than this amount. By doing so you may achieve equally good, or better results on the mental or emotional level, but purely physical effects may be diminished. This does not mean that the oil is not working well, and that the patient will not receive any benefit; it simply indicates that the effect is taking place on a higher, more subtle level. It is this kind of dose, and this kind of effect, that is involved in aromatherapy massage, or when using oils to spray the air of a treatment room.

At this point you may be wondering what is the point of extracting an oil from a plant, and then using it in such a small concentration that you could just as easily use the plant itself. Firstly, there are obvious practical reasons. Giving a back massage with a handful of sage leaves has its drawbacks. Secondly, the act of separating oil from a plant is equivalent to potentising a homoeopathic remedy: you are drawing out the more subtle nature of the plant. Braunschweig asks himself what is the point of distilling plants in order to make waters, when one could use the plant itself. His answer is 'to separate the grosse from subtil, and the subtil from the grosse'.

The path an essential oil takes in the body from ingestion to elimination varies. Some are eliminated through the lungs, some in the urine, a few through the skin, and many more via more than one path. Some are chemically changed in the body, and some are not. During their travels essences may partially lodge in the kidneys, liver, or other organ. The greater part of garlic oil, for instance, is eliminated through the lungs unchanged, and the rest via the urine. Most of sandalwood oil is eliminated with the urine, combined with glucuronic acid.

The effects of essences can be divided into two kinds: physiological and psychological. The former acts directly on the physical organism, the latter acts, via the sense of smell, on the mind, which in turn may cause a physiological effect. The second type of action is much less predictable than the first, and varies to some extent from person to person. It is discussed further in the following chapter.

Physiological effects can be subdivided into two types: those which act via the nervous system (and, perhaps, the endocrine system), and those which act directly on an organ or tissue. The two effects are quite distinct, although they may occur simultaneously. It is not always easy to ascertain which type of effect is taking place. The psychological effect can be ruled out when discussing experiments on animals, but even then it is not always certain whether the effect is nervous, or direct, or both. The words 'nervous', 'direct', and 'psychosomatic' are used to distinguish these three modes of action in the following text. The same action, e.g. antispasmodic, may be due in one instance to a nervous effect, and in another to a direct effect, according to the oil used.

In order to discuss the action of oils on the body in more detail I have found it most convenient to take each physiological system in turn. I have not included certain aspects of the action of essences which are self-evident, but have concentrated on those which I feel would be of particular interest.

The Digestive System

The first act of digestion is olfaction. The aroma of food stimulates the secretion of digestive juices, especially if it appeals to our sense of taste. The second act of digestion is tasting the food. This further stimulates the secretion of juices, especially saliva. Here it must be remembered that our taste buds can perceive only four basic flavours, and that the greater part of what we commonly call the taste of a food is in fact its smell. It is for this reason that food loses its taste when our nose is blocked.

The better our food tastes (and smells), the more we enjoy it and the better we digest it; hence the common use of spices and herbs in the kitchen. As with essences, so with herbs and spices: moderation produces the best results. If you take too many spicy foods you may overstrain your digestion and burden your kidneys; in moderation they aid digestion. All spices, and many herbs, encourage the flow of digestive juices, and discourage stomach spasms and flatulence. These properties are entirely due to the essential oils they contain.

The antispasmodic, carminative, and digestive actions of essences are well known, and many essences are still current in pharmacopoeias because of such properties. This subject formed the basis of a Japanese investigation carried out in 1963. Peppermint, fennel, cardamom, and several other essences were tested on excised mouse intestine. The investigators were not looking for the stimulation of digestive juice secretion so much as the acceleration of gastro-intestinal function and gas elimination. Such an acceleration was not observed to take place; indeed a very slight slowing down was noted in some cases. The oil did, however, show an antispasmodic action. The most interesting thing about this paper is the conclusion that the effect of essential oils on the human body is more likely to be a secondary effect via the olfactory and taste senses, rather than a direct one.

An Italian article, published in 1925, studied salivary secretion and the effects of essential oils on this secretion in man. It begins by establishing that the human secretion of saliva constantly oscillates between phases of secretion and non-secretion. This is independent of any external influences, such as those of smell. Under such influence the oscillation is still apparent, but takes place on a higher level, the secretion being more abundant. The essential oils of cloves, lavender, mint, and rosemary are shown to have a stimulating action on salivary secretion. This action takes place even when the nerve endings of the tongue are deadened, so that the sense of taste cannot operate. Results varied depending on whether they were pleasing or displeasing to the individual. This is obviously a psychosomatic effect. Smell appears to be more important than taste here.

This article only investigates the secretion of saliva, but the same may be true for the other digestive juices. As the Japanese article suggested, the digestive action of essential oils is primarily due to their effect via the sense of olfaction. However, the antispasmodic effect, which can be readily demonstrated on animals, would appear to be a direct physiological effect.

Several essences have a laxative effect. Their action is relatively mild, and takes the form of strengthening peristalsis (intestinal contractions). It is not clear whether the action is nervous or direct, although it would appear that at least some of the oils act via the nervous system. These oils include camphor, cinnamon, fennel, marjoram, and rosemary. They may be useful in constipation, flatulence, and lack of intestinal tone.

The opposite effect, that of reducing smooth muscle spasm, is observed in a large number of essences.[1] Thyme oil has the rare property of counteracting adrenaline spasm, and melissa, sage, and thyme are among those which reduce acetylcholine spasm. The action of melissa and sage is known to be nervous, while clary, clove, fennel, peppermint, rose, and thyme are considered to have a direct action. Clove oil counteracts stomach acidity by effectively raising the pH of gastric juice. Since this is due to its engenol content similar effects may be observed with oils of black pepper and cinnamon leaf.

Treatment for digestive disorders may be given orally, by enemas, by aromatic spinal massage, especially over the dorsal

1 See Antispasmodic p. 311.

and lumbar areas, and by local compresses over the stomach area or abdomen.

The Cardio-vascular System

This system comprises the heart, blood vessels, and spleen. The spleen is thought to be responsible for breaking down the worn-out red blood corpuscles. It also produces lymphocytes, and acts as a reservoir for blood. Under normal circumstances the spleen contracts rhythmically every twenty to thirty seconds. A number of factors influence the blood pressure, one of these being the contraction of the splenic blood vessels, and the spleen in general. Some oils, like calamus, cause dilation of the splenic vessels, thus producing a reduction of blood pressure. The action of calamus is interesting because it does not appear to be due to any nervous mechanism. As well as reducing blood pressure calamus reduces body temperature, and combats experimental auricular fibrillation in dogs. It appears to have an antispasmodic action on the heart, in common with oils of melissa and neroli. These oils may be used in palpitations, heart spasm, shock, etc.

Several other oils produce hypo- or hypertension by causing dilation or contraction of blood vessels. This action generally takes place via the autonomic nervous system. Camphor oil shows an opposite action to calamus, acting as a cardiac stimulant, vasco-constrictor, and increasing the blood pressure. The revival of the stopped heart by various agents succeeds better in camphor-treated frogs than in the controls, and the restored activity is more prolonged. Hyssop oil has a tonic action, causing first an increase, and then a decrease in blood pressure.

Some of the more yang oils stimulate the circulation, producing warmth and helping to raise the body temperature if it is low. These include benzoin, camphor, cinnamon, juniper, sage, and thyme. Oils of lavender and rose geranium produce arterial hypotension and a decrease in the surface tension of the blood, even in relatively small quantities.

Treatment may be given orally, by compresses over the heart area, by spinal massage, especially over the dorsal area, and by aromatic baths.

The Lymphatic System

As well as producing lymphocytes the spleen forms antibodies and antitoxins against infection. The lymphatic system is the waste-disposal system of the tissues, and it is largely in the lymph nodes that the battle against infection takes place. In an American study done in 1958 the *in vitro* antibacterial activity of 35 essential oils, 5 infused oils, and 95 combinations of these oils produced some interesting results. The oils were tested against five bacteria. None of the infused oils showed any antibacterial activity, and the addition of fatty oil to the essences greatly reduced their efficacy. The combinations consisted of mixtures of either two or three oils. Of the single essences the most effective were cinnamon, eucalyptus, and origanum. In general the essences were more effective against gram-positive than gram-negative bacteria. Of the 47 combinations of two essences none were found to enhance antibacterial activity; in fact 45 of the combinations showed a decrease in activity. Of the 15 combinations of three oils, 3 of these combinations were found to exhibit greater antibacterial activity than each essence used separately.

It would seem, judging by the above information, that if essences were being used as antibacterial agents they should not be diluted in vegetable oils. At the same time, if we blend essences to use against infection we may actually be reducing their antibacterial potency, and so it would seem wiser to use a single essence that we know to be effective.

On the other hand clinical results are more conclusive than *in vitro* tests. I have treated many throat infections, a few of them chronic, by the external application of essential oils diluted in either water or oil. In most cases a rapid and positive result was obtained. It is not clear whether the diluted essences did perform an antibacterial role, or whether they acted by somehow enhancing the natural defence mechanisms of the body. The often dynamic results achieved lead one to suspect that both may be taking place at the same time.

Essential oils in general are in fact known to stimulate leucocytosis. Rovesti (1971) talks of 'recent experiments of considerable importance regarding the stimulating action, and the increase of white blood corpuscles caused by essences in general, of which lavender has turned out to be one of the most effective. As with bergamot and lemon, *this occurs either through inhalation or cutaneous absorption as well as orally.*' He mentions that this mechanism of stimulating organic defence was known to Kobert at the turn of the century; and to Benedicenti, one of

Rovesti's more recent predecessors: 'Benedicenti foresaw preparations based on essences of bergamot, lavender and lemon to stimulate a "curative leucocytosis" in various types of infection.'

An article by Y. Ruckebusch and H. M. Gattefossé (1964) talks of the 'phagocytic' power of essential oils, meaning their power to stimulate phagocytosis: 'This phagocytic property is found in all essences which, applied to a purulent, traumatised, or healthy skin, bring about a rapid disappearance of related (microbial) phenomena and a total cicatrisation'. The authors mention that all essences have this property to varying degrees, in particular oil of terebinth.

Dr Valnet mentions three essences (camomile, lemon, thyme) as being stimulants of leucocytosis. Okanishi (1928) refers to oils of pine needle, sandlewood, and vetivert in this context.

It is clear that essential oils, as well as being powerful antiseptics, have the ability to stimulate the natural defences of the body against infection. In this they are useful as prophylactic agents, helping to prevent infection in cases of epidemic. They would thus be invaluable as air purifiers in hospitals, and were used as such in some French hospitals and schools in the earlier part of this century. Essences in general stimulate both leucocytosis and phagocytosis. Although some oils are more generally effective (bergamot, lavender, etc.) it may be that certain oils work better for certain people, depending on their state of physical and mental health.

The Respiratory System

The antiseptic, antispasmodic, and expectorant action of essential oils is of interest here. As antiseptics they may be used in all types of respiratory infection. For general use oils of bergamot, cinnamon, and eucalyptus are most valuable. Bergamot oil is effective against the diphtheria bacillus, as is garlic oil, and camphor oil has proved successful in pneumococcus infections, such as pneumonia. There are a number of influenza viruses. In 1973 a Russian study showed that certain eucalyptus oils were effective *in vitro* against influenza viruses A_2 and A. For general use in influenza cinnamon, eucalyptus, or black pepper are most useful.

A study on the antispasmodic properties of essential oils including clary, fennel, peppermint, rose, and thyme was carried out in 1968 in Bulgaria. All the oils showed an antispasmodic effect on smooth muscle at concentration of 50 – 100 γ/ml; concentrations of less than 10 γ/ml were ineffective. A 5% dilution of essences from clary and thyme was found to increase the respiratory volume and decrease the blood pressure. The Antispasmodic effect is considered to be chiefly direct.

Camphor oil has been found to be a general respiratory stimulant, increasing both the rate and amplitude of respiration.

In 1946 a study on the expectorant action of certain essential oils was carried out by two Canadians, E. M. Boyd and G. L. Pearson. The oils included eucalyptus and lemon, and were given by stomach tube to guinea pigs. They were found to increase the output of respiratory tract fluid. The most effective dose was 50 mg/kg of body weight, which is equivalent to an adult human of 150 lb taking 3.4 grams of essence. This is a very high dose. The expectorant action was shown to be direct rather than nervous.

Boyd, this time in collaboration with E. P. Sheppard, published the results of a similar study in 1968. It showed that eucalyptus oil produced a dose-dependent increase in the output of respiratory tract fluid. Doses sufficient to produce a satisfactory secretion were also so large that local inflammation of the mucous membrane was produced.

In 1970 Boyd and Sheppard gave lemon oil by steam inhalation to rabbits. It was found to increase the volume output of respiratory tract fluid, and to increase its mucus concentration. The action appeared to be due to a local secretion of the secretory cells, and was thus direct. The dosage used in this experiment is interesting, and quite different from that used in the previous two studies. The amount given was just below that which imparted a perceptible odour of lemon to the inhaled air, and was equivalent to 0.00068 grams for an adult human of 150 lb. This is equal to approximately one-thirtieth of a drop of lemon oil. When the dosage of lemon oil was increased to perceptible amounts the expectorant action declined.

The 1946 experiment, which included lemon oil, concluded that a very large dose was necessary, and that amounts below this were much less effective. The 1970 study concluded that an extremely small dose of lemon oil was also effective, and that larger amounts were ineffective. The only important difference in these studies is that in the earlier one oils were given by stomach tube, and they were given by steam inhalation in 1970.

However, in the 1968 study the oils were also given by steam inhalation, and the results for large doses were similar to those for the 1946 study. It can only be assumed that what we are seeing here is something like a homoeopathic phenomenon, where very small amounts are equally effective as large amounts.

Essential oils for respiratory complaints may be given orally, by inhalation, by spinal massage, especially to the cervical or dorsal area, or by local compresses.

The Urinary System

Oils of juniper, sage, sandalwood, and thyme are effective against urinary tract infection with staphylococcus aureus. The same oils, plus camphor oil, are good diuretics. Juniper oil acts by enhancing glomerular filtration, and also produces an increase in the amounts of potassium, sodium, and chlorine excreted. In rabbits with experimental glomeronephritis, the high blood urea levels were reduced by an aqueous solution of camomile oil given by stomach tube. Gatti and Cajola report that sandalwood is effective in haematuria caused by renal malfunction. A number of essences, especially camomile and geranium, effectively dissolve urinary stones.

Treatment with essences may be given orally, by hip baths, lumbo-sacral massage, or local compress.

The Reproductive System

In 1974 there were 750,000 known cases of gonorrhoea in the USA. In 1930 Collier and Nitta found that bergamot oil was effective against gonococcus in a dilution of 1:600. Although sandalwood oil does not appear to be effective against gonococcus it is nevertheless very useful in treating gonorrhoea.[1] An antibacterial agent is not necessarily needed in order to cure an infection.

The way emmenagoguic essences affect the body is not clear. Oils of Pennyroyal and savin (which have a very strong action, but are also highly toxic) have been found to have no stimulating action on the excised uterus; in fact they were found to inhibit contractions. It has been suggested that their action is due to constitutional poisoning or gastro-intestinal irritation. However, this would not explain their efficacy when applied externally, or in

1 See sandalwood, p. 285.

relatively small doses. It seems more likely that the effect takes place via the nervous system, or perhaps is due to an indirect hormonal effect.

Linked to their emmenagoguic effect is the parturient, or oxytocic, action of certain oils, that is to say they help to induce labour by stimulating uterine contraction, and may help to give a swift and relatively painless birth. Such oils include jasmine and juniper. The use of organic agents for this purpose is preferable in some cases to drugs or hormones, since they are much safer, and encourage a natural birth instead of a forced, often over-hurried affair. Synthetic oxytocin, which is most commonly used to induce labour, can produce such strong contractions that the mother is caused a great deal of pain — in which case a pain-killing drug is usually given. The baby has to suffer the unnaturally strong contractions, and is often born much quicker than normal. Both these factors contribute to increasing the already traumatic effect of birth for the baby. The pain-killer, usually pethidine, causes the baby to be born already doped, and many of these babies show a very low degree of alertness in the early years of their life. Breast feeding is usually difficult to establish, and the mother-child relationship may be permanently affected.

During an induction the effects on the baby are constantly monitored, and it if reacts adversely an emergency caesarian is usually necessary. After the birth another drug is usually given to bring out the afterbirth. What really amazes me is that hospitalisation is now expected for the great majority of births, and that births are induced simply so that they will occur at a time of day convenient to the hospital staff. How far away from nature can one get?

Parturient oils may be applied in compresses to the lower abdomen or massage to the lower back; they may also be taken orally.

Many aromatics, usually the more stimulating ones, are reputed to be aphrodisiacs, although I know of no clinical studies on this subject. The usual definition of aphrodisiac is a drug which increases sexual desire, although it is also mentioned with reference to increasing sexual stamina and performance. Obviously the two are to some extent linked, but a lack of one factor is possible without a lack of the other. Notable aphrodisiacs are jasmine, and ylang-ylang. Obviously the scent is an important factor here; most cases of impotence or frigidity are found to be related to psychological problems.

For problems of the reproductive system oils may be used orally, in massage, hip baths, or vaginal douches.

The Endocrine System

There are two basic ways in which essential oils affect the endocrine function. Firstly, they may stimulate certain glands, thus stimulating or normalising hormonal secretion. Secondly they may act as quasi-hormones themselves. Dr Valnet cites oils of basil, geranium, pine, rosemary, and sage as being adrenal cortex stimulants. Gattefossé comments: 'It is now known that mint stimulates the hypophyseal secretions.' Jasmine may have a similar influence. I have been unable to trace any further evidence of glandular stimulation, although I feel sure that all the endocrine glands are affected by one or more essences, whether directly or indirectly. The pronounced effect of aromatic oils on the emotions, their aphrodisiac effect, and their action on the nervous system would seem to indicate endocrine influence.

Plant hormones, or phytohormones, have recently caught the interest of manufacturers of natural cosmetics, because of their effect on the skin. Hormone creams, which contain animal hormones, have been used for many years for their rejuvenating effect, but occasionally these hormones have unfortunate side-effects on the body; excessive use of these creams has been known to cause unsightly puffiness of the skin. Phytohormones seem to offer a more versatile and safer alternative. They also have the advantage of not being shunned by those who prefer to avoid cosmetics which contain animal-derived ingredients.

Phytohormones are generally regarded today as substances found in plants which chemically resemble animal hormones. Their possible use in therapy has not yet been seriously considered, and little is known of their physiological effects, in comparison with animal hormones. Sometimes phytohormones are contained in the essential oil of a plant: they are found in pollen extracts, eucalyptus, fennel, hops, dandelion, garlic, licorice root, sarsaparilla, ginseng, and many other plants. Sarsaparilla contains testosterone, vitex agnus castus has an effect resembling that of progesterone, and hops are rich in oestrogen. Significant disturbances of fertility sometimes occur in grazing animals which consume large amounts of certain herbs. Female hop-pickers may suffer disturbances of their menstrual cycle.

Many plants contain oestrogens. Oestriole or oestrone have been found in the catkins of willow trees, and folliculin is present in garlic, ginseng, hops, licorice root, and oats. Oestrogenic activity has been demonstrated by essential oils of aniseed, fennel, and to a slight extent eucalyptus; aniseed and fennel have been used as galactagogues since ancient times. Most of the phytohormone-containing plants are aromatic. Although the phytohormones are not always present in the essence it is possible that the latter still has some hormonal activity. Jasmine oil has not been investigated, but would appear to have a strong hormonal influence.

Gattefossé mentions plant hormones in a slightly different light, and is not so eager to compare them with animal hormones. He attributes the discovery and identification of phytohormones to a certain Gavrilovitch, who classified them into three categories:

1. Male and female floral (sexual) hormones
2. Embryonic (germinative) hormones
3. Growth hormones

These hormones are said to be present particularly in plants containing very apparent reproductive organs. Gattefossé demonstrated the interdependence of these hormones (which may be compared to the interdependence of hormones in animals). When the sexual hormone is at its strongest, for instance, the potential of the other hormones is considerably reduced, and vice versa: the total hormonal potential is maintained at a constant level. Plant hormones are also interdependent for another reason; the germinative hormones actually give rise to the growth hormones, which give rise to the sexual hormones, which in turn give rise to the germinative hormones. Thus a continual hormonal cycle takes place, which may itself be regulated by an as yet unknown hormone. Could this 'unknown hormone' in fact be the essential oil?

Speaking of their effect on the skin, Gattefossé says:

> 'Extremely active, whether applied via the skin or mucous membrane, they provoke a remarkable firming of the skin, stimulate the metabolism of the dermal cells and act as a rejuvenating active principle.

Floral hormones regulate sebaceous secretions and act with the same efficacy in the two opposite cases: dry skin and oily skin.'

The subject of phytohormones is a fascinating one, and merits a great deal more research than has so far been devoted to it. Endocrine disturbance is manifested in virtually every type of disease, and the possibility of treating it directly with plant extracts or essential oils is, to say the least, interesting. Although essences do not always contain hormones, it would appear that many of them have a hormone-regulating effect, which may in some cases be more useful than the direct use of phytohormones themselves.

In conclusion I would like to mention a German study of milk secretion in goats. (Milk secretion is only directly influenced by hormones, although other factors may have an indirect effect.) The effects of fennel oil, common salt, arsenic, and the visual effect of grass were studied. It was found that salt and fennel oil had a favourable influence on both the total quantity of milk, and its fat content. Arsenic and the visual effect of grass had practically no effect. The author of this paper, G. Fingerling, believes that either odour or taste is necessary to influence lacteal secretion.

The Nervous System

It is difficult to classify essences according to their action on the nervous system because there is very little detailed information on the subject, and so far nobody appears to have made a comprehensive study. Also many essences have both stimulating and sedative properties, and to classify an essential oil as simply 'stimulant' or 'sedative' can be misleading and confusing. Unfortunately the use of these two words is unavoidable in a discussion such as this.

The old herbalists classified most aromatics as hot and dry, and aromatics are traditionally thought of as stimulating. They were often prescribed in nervous disorders such as 'falling sickness', melancholy, and paralysis. In ancient times aromatics were used to drive evil spirits out of people who were in fact suffering from some form of nervous or emotional disturbance.

Gatti and Cajola classified oils as basically stimulating or sedative. Among the first group they included oils of cedar, cardamom, fennel, cinnamon, lemon, and ylang-ylang; in the second oils of cajuput, camomile, melissa, and peppermint. Later studies have shown that peppermint oil is stupefying in large doses, although small amounts have more of a stimulating action.

Stimulating aromatics were traditionally used for states of depression, languor, and disorders associated with lack of nerve function such as paralysis, loss of voice, etc. They were also used for any condition associated with coldness. Although this usually applied to physical coldness it could equally well refer to emotional coldness. Many aromatics, especially rosemary, were said to be good for loss of memory and mental weakness. Daniel McKenzie suggests that this is due to the action of certain smells in reminding us of past events. However, it refers rather to rousing a weak memory, and general mental weakness (inability to concentrate, etc.), by a stimulating action on the brain. This is what was meant by the word 'cephalic' (literally, 'of the head'), although this word was also used to refer to physical disorders of the head.

As sedatives essences were used for hysteria, insomnia, and states of nervousness, an action which several modern studies confirm; 'camomile . . . oil decreased the spontaneous activity of mice' (Kudrzycka-Bieloszabska, 1966); 'In experiments with 126 mice, a study was made of motor activity, the position of the eyelids and the general state after the i.p. [Intraperitoneal] injection of a 5% emulsion of essential oils . . . general depression without ataraxia was observed' (Shipochliev, 1968). The oils used in this last study include basil, clary, sage, fennel, geranium, marjoram, and rose. A study of the effects of marjoram on the autonomic nervous system (Caujolle and Franck, 1945) had the following results:

> '[Parasympathetic effects] The oil, injected intra-
> venously, increases the cardiomoderator effect of com-
> pression of the eyeballs, and increases the vasodilator
> effect of electrical stimulation of Hering's nerve. Sym-
> pathetic effects: it decreases the hypertensive effect of
> temporary occlusion of the main carotid arteries after
> section of the depressor nerves, decreases the
> vasoconstrictor action of adrenaline, and increases the
> vasodilator and cardiomoderator effects of
> acetylcholine.'

Studies on oils of lavender and melissa have revealed a pronounced sedative action. The effect of melissa is referred to as narcotic.

According to Cadéac and Meunier melissa and peppermint are stupefying in large doses.

Lesieur classified essences into three main groups: convulsive, excito-stupefying, and stupefying. In the first group he includes oils of hyssop and rosemary, in the third group melissa and thyme. He subdivides the second group into oils which are primarily stimulant (peppermint) and those which are primarily sedative (basil, marjoram). The convulsive group can cause epileptic fits, but only in people predisposed to epilepsy. According to Dr Valnet this group includes essential oils of rosemary, fennel, hyssop, sage (but not clary), and wormwood. However, I would not include oils of fennel and rosemary in such a group. Some essences are anti-convulsive, although the therapeutic value of these oils has yet to be proved; they include calamus, clary sage, and lavender, which have proved effective against electrical shock convulsions. It may be that one or more of these oils is of use in the treatment of epilepsy.

From my own experience clary sage oil has a very pronounced effect on the nervous system, even in small doses.[1] Similar effects to that of clary may be obtained by other oils, notably jasmine. Oil of nutmeg contains phenylpropenes similar in structure to mescaline (elemicin and myristicin). In large doses (7 – 12 g) it is stupefying, and produces symptoms similar to alcohol poisoning (delirium, hallucinations, stupor, loss of memory). In these amounts nutmeg oil is highly toxic, and should never be taken, especially by epileptics. Further information on the use of essences in psychological disturbance is given in the following chapter.

1 See clary sage, p. 210.

Chapter 6

The Mind

'Physicians might (in my opinion) draw more use and good from odours than they do. For myself have often perceived, that according unto their strength and qualitie, they change, and alter, and move my spirit, and worke strange effects in me: Which makes me approve the common saying that invention of incense and perfumes in Churches, so ancient and so far-dispersed throughout all nations and religions, had an especiall regard to rejoyce, to comfort, to quicken and to rowze and to purifie our senses.'

Montaigne

'Disease is in essence the result of conflict between soul and Mind. . . . So long as our Souls and personalities are in harmony all is joy and peace, happiness and health. It is when our personalities are led astray from the path laid down by the Soul, either by our own worldly desires or by the persuasion of others, that a conflict arises.'

Edward Bach

Quite naturally we tend to think of *mind* and *body* as two separate entities. The body exists and functions on the physical plane, and the mind simply thinks. However, although we may not always be aware of it, mind and body are constantly inter-reacting on the deepest of levels. We have an interesting word, *psychosomatic*, which means 'having both mental and physical elements'; a condition which is emotional in origin, but also has a physical manifestation. Medical science is coming to realise more and more how important this branch of therapeutics is. Many physical conditions, such as asthma and colitis, are now recognised as having a strong psychosomatic element.

The fact that our mental state affects our physical state is hardly surprising if we see people as one entity in the first place. At the same time let us not be blind to the fact that our mind and our body are not the same thing at all. Our body is purely physical; after death it remains. Our mind is non-physical, though it manifests itself through our body; it does not remain after death. However, the two closely interact, the one affecting the other. There is also a third element, the soul, which is neither mind not body. It is that consciousness which is there when we are born, before our mind has begun to develop. It is the 'I' in us, the one constant throughout our lives. It is non-physical, neither does it think, but it feels and 'experiences'.

Our mind affects our body primarily through the autonomic nervous system, and the glands regulated by the autonomic nerves may be overstimulated. They may, for example, trigger excessive secretion of gastric juices which, in time, may erode the lining of the stomach or jejunum, causing a peptic ulcer. Cramp, diarrhoea, constipation, indigestion, and many other disorders may be psychosomatic. Many people feel embarrassed at the thought that their body is being affected by their mind. We feel embarrassed because we cannot do anything about it, and yet we are causing our own distress. We seem to be at the mercy of our mind and our emotions. But if we are at the mercy of our mind, even embarrassed by it, what are *we*? What is feeling embarrassed? It is not mind or body, but soul. Feelings come from our soul as well as our mind, and are very often produced by a mind-soul relationship.

Our soul is the life force within us; it gives life to the body. When we experience peace of mind the soul is able to shine through. Its attributes are positive ones: generosity, love, selflessness, warmth. Unfortunately we also have a negative aspect which tends to predominate and which, for the sake of argument, we can call the mind. It is this aspect which gives rise to selfish desires, fears and hatred.

Because most of us think we are our mind (that which thinks) rather than our soul (that which is the very life within us and

gives mind the energy to think) we become confused, and sometimes depressed. Our mind seems to have an excess of energy; it
thinks even when it is not required to, giving rise to all kinds of
anxieties. By associating ourselves with the soul, and with the
positive attributes of love and selflessness, we can greatly limit
the negative aspects of the mind which lead to physical and
mental disease. Dr Edward Bach, a physician of great spiritual
insight, wrote about this very problem:

'Pride, which is arrogance and rigidity of mind, will give
rise to those diseases which produce rigidity and stiffness
of the body. Pain is the result of cruelty, whereby the
patient learns through personal suffering not to inflict it
upon others, either from a physical or from a mental
standpoint. The penalties of Hate are loneliness, violent
uncontrollable temper, mental nerve storms and conditions of hysteria. The disease of introspection —
neurosis, neurasthenia and similar conditions — which
rob life of so much enjoyment, are caused by excessive
Self-love. Ignorance and lack of wisdom bring their own
difficulties in everyday life, and in addition should there
be a persistence in refusing to see truth when the oppor-
tunity has been given, short-sightedness and impairment
of vision and hearing are the natural consequences.
Instability of mind must lead to the same quality in the
body with those various disorders which affect movement and co-ordination. The result of greed and
domination of others is such diseases as will render the
sufferer a slave to his own body, with desires and ambi-
tions curbed by the malady.

'Moveover, the very part of the body affected is no
accident, but is in accordance with the law of cause and
effect, and again will be a guide to help us. For
example, the heart, the fountain of life and hence of
love, is attacked when especially the love side of the
nature towards humanity is not developed or is wrongly
used; a hand affected denotes failure or wrong in action;
the brain being the centre of control, if afflicted,
indicates lack of control in the personality. Such must
follow as the law lays down. We are all ready to admit
the many results which may follow a fit of violent

temper, the shock of sudden bad news; if trivial affairs can thus affect the body, how much more serious and deep-rooted must be a prolonged conflict between soul and body. Can we wonder that the result gives rise to such grievous complaints as the diseases amongst us today?'

Edward Bach sees the first duty of the physician as one of inspiration and spiritual guidance, to help us to heal ourselves by seeing where we have gone wrong. He continues:

'The second duty of the physician will be to administer such remedies as will help the physical body to gain strength and assist the mind to become calm, widen its outlook and strive towards perfection, thus bringing peace and harmony to the whole personality. Such remedies there are in nature, placed there by the mercy of the Divine Creator for the healing and comfort of mankind.'

Essences can be of use as therapeutic agents in a similar way to ordinary tranquillisers, although they work organically, and in a more subtle way. Aromatics have been used for states of emotional disturbance from the times when they were first used as incense. Part of the reason for the worldwide popularity of incense in religious ceremony may be its effect on the mind. Generally speaking, essences have an uplifting, and at the same time calming, effect, as many old herbals testify:

'Artemisia. To make a child mery hange a bondell of mugwort or make smoke thereof under the chylde's bedde for it taketh away annoy for hem.'

'Also drye roses put to ye nose to smell do conforte the braine and the harte.'

'Bawme comforts the heart and driveth away all melancholy and sadnesse.'

Perhaps this last comment is somewhat optimistic, but we can see that aromatic herbs have been used in this connection for a long time. Leading physicians of antiquity such as Galen and Celsus advocated the use of aromatic herbs as sovereign remedies against hysterical convulsions, and report that they sometimes stopped attacks immediately. Unlike the modern sleeping pill, essences are not mere sedatives; most of them are very pleasant to smell — hence the uplifting effect. Madame Marguerite Maury had this to say:

> 'But of the greatest interest is the effect of the fragrance on the psychic and mental state of the individual. Powers of perception become clearer and more acute, and there is a feeling of having seen more objectively and therefore in truer perspective. It might even be said that the emotional trouble which in general obscures our perception is practically suppressed.'

Here she is talking about the effect which I have termed 'uplifting', where the essence raises us above our problems, making us feel lighter and more detached. Depression, despair, and other negative feelings always make us feel heavy, and they stem from desires and fears of the mind. Joy is a light feeling, and comes directly from the soul. Although they work through the sense of smell essences go deeper than the senses. They work on our mind, lightening it, making it less heavy, less dark. Although essences cannot liberate our souls they can, by lightening the mind, help the light of the soul to shine through.

At the same time as they uplift our spirits they have a calming effect on the nervous system. The very nervous person, with his constipation or peptic ulcer, finds it easier to relax, and, as essences are relatively mild sedatives, there is no danger of side-effects.

As long as we realise the limitations of all such therapeutic agents, we will put them to the best possible use. Even essences are, after all, only a crutch. If all that was necessary to get rid of our emotional problems was for us to take something uplifting, or sedative, or both, then we might do as well with hashish, LSD, heroin, and the like. But essences are safer crutches. They are effective without being dangerous; subtle, but not so subtle that there is no apparent effect.

Professor Rovesti has been studying the effects of essences on the psyche. He comments:

> 'According to sociologists and neurologists the salient characteristics of our age are those of anxiety and

depression, and material proof of this is available in the even higher figures shown for the consumption of tranquillisers and stimulants. It is well known that disturbance and toxicosis can be caused by these products if taken regularly.

'Both neuroses often cause aversion to any type of pleasure, by producing a sense of weariness which many people are unable to overcome.

'The possibility of applying new therapies to these widespread psycho-neuroses is therefore of considerable importance.

'For such purposes, therefore, interest attaches to the use of essential oils as aids, or even as sole remedies in psychotherapy.

'The matter is of still further interest, since the essential oils that are employed in aromatherapy, in the appropriate doses, are harmless to the organism and do not cause troubles like those produced by the ordinary psychological drugs. Very conclusive experiments in this direction have been carried out in various clinics for nervous diseases, on patients affected by hysteria or psychic depression.'

Rovesti does not suggest that essences can take the place of psychotherapy in its many and varied forms, but that they form a useful and safer adjunct to such therapies than chemical tranquillisers. Let me emphasise here that, in the case of serious mental disturbance, essences cannot be expected to do the whole job on their own: they are not miracle drugs. In such cases some form of counselling, psychotherapy or spiritual inspiration is needed in combination with aromatherapy. In the same way a purely physical treatment with essences is greatly enhanced by massage, diet, or some other form of natural therapy.

Drs Gatti and Cajola made some studies of the effects of essential oils on the nervous system. They noted the two basic types of emotional disturbance: one over-excited, tense, talkative, anxious and the other melancholic, apathetic, silent. They also noted that a number of essences were either nerve stimulants or nerve sedatives, and that the traditional 'cephalic' or 'nervine' herbs were usually aromatic. They found that camomile and melissa were antispasmodics and nerve sedatives, and that ylang-ylang was a mild nerve stimulant and had an aphrodisiac effect. They also found that oils of geranium and patchouli were effective in states of tension and anxiety. They applied the essences by spraying the surrounding air, or by giving the patients cotton wool to sniff, impregnated with oils.

Rovesti has found the former method successful, and also observes that 'by placing on a lump of sugar one to three drops of the essential oils referred to and by keeping this on the tongue without swallowing it, so as to cause it to dissolve slowly, producing a respiratory inhalation of essential oil vapours, at least three times a day, the degree of anxiety and nervous excitability was considerably lowered'. The essential oils referred to include bergamot, camphor, cypress, lavender, marjoram, neroli, and rose. One might add that the use of essences in baths or massage is equally effective, and that there are two important factors to consider here. First, the essences have a *dual* action; that of smelling a pleasant perfume, or flower (which, by the very fact that it smell appealing, attracts and soothes the mind), and that of a nerve sedative or stimulant, which acts independently of the sense of smell. Secondly, if essences are to have their full effect on the mind perception by smell must take place. Through the sense of smell essences have a direct and rapid effect on the mind. They are so highly aromatic that it is difficult to use them without olfaction taking place.

If part of the psychological effect of oils is due to their odour, as perceived by the individual, we cannot expect them to have their full effect if they are perceived as unpleasant. We may, therefore, expect to find that the most universally pleasing oils, such as jasmine and rose, have the greatest potential in this type of therapy, and that the oil most pleasing to an individual may have the most pronounced therapeutic effect. Rovesti mentions that blends of essences, which can produce more pleasing scents than individual oils, are often more pleasant and acceptable to the patient. Blends may contain oils which, on their own, are not attractive, but in combination with others produce a satisfactory result.

For the treatment of depressive states Rovesti recommends oils of citrus fruits, ylang-ylang, and compositions based on sandalwood, patchouli, jasmine, and cloves. One may also mention basil and peppermint here, which have a similar refreshing and uplifting effect to citrus oils. Some oils, notably bergamot, lavender, and geranium, have proved useful in both anxiety (nervous tension) and depression. This demonstrates the versatility of essences as therapeutic agents, and their ability to respond to the needs of the individual. Not everybody can be neatly slotted into the states of either 'anxiety' or 'depression'. Sometimes the characteristics of the two states are mixed, or alternate with moods of feverish activity, followed by depression. We can see the same 'human element' in essential oils, which cannot be classified simply as stimulating or sedative. Their action is more complex and subtle than this. Rovesti comments:

> 'It is obviously not possible to define precise limits between the two aroma-therapeutic actions of nerve stimulants and nerve sedatives, not only because of the complexity of the composition of essential oils (which in most cases contain various types of osmophoric functions) but moreover because of their particular type of general physiological action, which Kobert has defined as simultaneously both stimulating and sedative. Whereas in fact in some substances factors are involved that are mainly exciting or sedative, in others (and these are in the majority) the two pharmacological actions are mixed, so that in certain doses they are stimulants and in others sedatives.'

One is reminded of the organic nature of essences, and of their ability to adapt, normalise, or balance rather than simply stimulate or sedate. Their action, as I have suggested, is more complex and subtle, because each essence has an affinity with certain parts of the body, certain areas of the mind, and certain types of emotion. Just as someone with a hard heart may develop heart disease, or hardening of the arteries, so the essences which relieve the physical condition may also act on the mental state. To summarise:

Anxiety, nervous tension benzoin, bergamot, camomile, camphor, cypress, geranium, jasmine, lavender, marjoram, melissa, neroli, rose, sandalwood, ylang-ylang

Depression, melancholy	basil, bergamot, camomile, frankincense, geranium, jasmine, lavender, neroli, patchouli, peppermint, rose, sandalwood, ylang-ylang

This is a useful guide for treating anxiety and depression, but most physical ailments also involve a psychological factor. This factor may or may not be the cause of the disease, but it is unwise to ignore it completely. To give a more precise, individual treatment it is necessary to be clear about the psychological state of the individual, who may be depressed because of other emotions, such as fear or guilt. In order to treat a variety of mental states we need to know more about the action of essences on the mind. As a guide I have compiled the following table, which is largely based on my own experience.

Anger	camomile, melissa, rose, ylang-ylang
Apathy	jasmine, juniper, patchouli, rosemary
Confusion, indecision	basil, cypress, frankincense, peppermint, patchouli
Dwelling on unpleasant past events	benzoin, frankincense
Fear, paranoia	basil, clary, jasmine, juniper
Grief	hyssop, marjoram, rose
Hypersensitivity	camomile, jasmine, melissa
Hypochrondria	jasmine, melissa
Impatience, irritability	camomile, camphor, cypress, lavender, marjoram, frankincense
Jealousy	rose
Panic, hysteria	camomile, clary, jasmine, lavender, marjoram, melissa, neroli, ylang-ylang
Shock	camphor, melissa, neroli
Suspicion	lavender

The purpose of this table is to indicate the action of aromatic oils on the mind so that you will be able to choose more wisely for each individual treated. Essences will obviously be more effective when the physical symptoms correlate with the mental syndrome. If you are treating someone whose problem seems to be largely psychological in origin the choice of essences to suit their mental state will be of prime importance. I am aware that there are several states of mind not included in the above table. In this case I advise you to choose the nearest mental aspect to the one in question; for example in the case of hate, consult the oils for anger, in the case of resentment consult jealousy. I have purposely kept the table short and concise because the qualities given have not been widely tried and tested. For the same reason I have not included them in the Therapeutic Index.

The more you use essences, and the more you get to know them, the more you will see how they act on the mind and what their individual qualities are. Each essence has its own personality, its own set of attributes, and this can be used to bring out certain qualities in us; helping us to see ourselves more clearly, to understand our faults, and to let the beauty and joy of our souls breath a fresh, summery fragrance through our minds.

Chapter 7

Aromatic Baths

'Here first she bathes, and round her body pours
Soft oils of fragrance and ambrosial showers,
The winds, perfumed, the balmy gale conveys
Through heaven, through earth, and all the aerial ways.'

Homer

Bathing has always been popular whether for enjoyment, health, or hygiene. It seems to have been more often associated with aromatics than with water, if we define bathing as a process of cleansing the body. Whenever bathing with water was unfashionable or impractical, aromatics were used to cleanse or perfume the skin. When bathing with water was employed aromatics were never far away, being used either as scented bath oils, or as scented massage oils after bathing. In either case they would act as antiseptics, improving the hygienic value of bathing and helping to reduce body odour.

The ancient Egyptians, particularly the women (at least, those who were able to afford it), showed their high degree of civilisation by an extraordinarily refined use of the bath. Every day they would take a succession of baths; first cold, then tepid, and then hot. The hot bath, which was scented with fragrant oils, was followed by an aromatic massage, probably with cedar-wood oil or cypress. This, and the other elaborate rituals of their toilet (hairdressing, face massage, facial and breast make-up), was attended to by slaves.

The ancient Syrians also enjoyed bathing, and had public baths. Eugene Rimmel relates the story of a Syrian king, who went by the name of Antiochus. The story goes that this king was once bathing in the public baths, with all his slaves in attendance, when he was approached by one of the common people. 'You are a happy man, O King,' he said, 'you smell in a most costly manner.' At this the king was very pleased, and replied: 'I will give you as much as you can desire of this perfume.' He then ordered a larger ewer of thick, aromatic unguent to be poured over the man's head, and the area was soon crowded with commoners, jostling for some of the expensive perfume. This caused the king infinite amusement, but as he turned to go he slipped on the expensive unguent, and fell on his back.

Although the Egyptian system of bathing was partly adopted by the Greeks, they never gave it that elaborate development which it acquired afterwards with the Romans. The Greek male was usually satisfied with more limited ablutions, performed in a marble basin situated in some public place. Women, of course, always attended to their toilet in the privacy of their own home.

The Romans must have been the greatest bathers of all time. Like the Egyptians they had public baths, which were extremely popular with the men, women usually preferring to bath at home. The baths, or *thermae*, formed one of the most important features of the Roman social life. The principal baths were magnificent buildings, and were erected by various emperors, perhaps the finest being built by the Emperor Caracalla in the third century AD. At one time there were almost a thousand public baths in Rome.

On entering a Roman bath one first undressed and then entered a room called the *unctuarium*, which had shelf upon shelf of terracotta jars containing perfumes and fragrant ointments. Having received a preliminary oiling one proceeded to the *frigidarium*, or cold bath, for a quick, stimulating rubdown. Next came the *tepidarium*, or tepid bath, and then the *caldarium*, the hot bath, which was heated by a furnace underneath called the *hypocaustum*, the predecessor of our modern steam bath. While in the hot bath one scrubbed oneself all over with a sort of bronze curry-comb called a 'strigil', at the same time pouring scented oil over the body from a small bottle, an *ampulla*. After the hot bath came a relaxing massage with fragrant oils. Those who could afford it had all these duties performed either by the bath attendants or by their own slaves.

Roman women were usually attended to at home; the wealthy had several slaves for this purpose, in the style of the Egyptians.

They were known as *cosmetae*, and were overseen by the *orna-trix*, the mistress of the toilet. After bathing, the hair was styled, dyed, and treated with fragrant oils. The face was then massaged, the cheeks painted with *fucus*, a kind of rouge, and the eyes shaded. Finally the neck and shoulders were massaged with scented oils, and the rest of the body lightly washed in rose water.

We now turn from the sophistication of ancient Egypt and Rome to more recent times, and more perfunctory circumstances. In certain parts of the world, especially in the African continent, water is scarce, and bathing in it impractical. I quote from Eugene Rimmel:

> 'There is a very curious sort of bath used in Nubia which deserves particular description. Consul Petherick relates that, having ordered a *bath* at Berbera, one of the Nubian towns he visited, he was much surprised at seeing a negro maid enter bearing a bowl and a teacup as the sole apparatus required. The bowl contained dough, and the cup a small quantity of sweet oil scented with aromatic roots; the former of these well rubbed on the bare skin cleaned it thoroughly, after which the perfumed oil was applied, to give elasticity to the limbs. The whole operation, which is called "dilka", is in great favour with the natives; and Mr Petherick, who declares he was much refreshed by it, attributes to its use the entire absence of cutaneous disease among these people, and says it enables them to resist the cold and cutting winds of winter with no other protection than very thin clothing.
>
> 'An aromatic fumigation replaces, in the Soudan, even this very imperfect mode of bathing. In a hole, dug in the ground by the side of the bed, is placed an earthen pot, in which is burned the odoriferous wood of the tulloch. The natives sit over this, covering themselves closely with a thick woollen wrapper, and remain exposed for about ten minutes to the cloud of fragrant smoke, which causes intense perspiration, and is supposed to exercise a tonic and beneficial influence on the skin.'

This also bears a very strong resemblance to our modern steam bath.

In Europe bathing was introduced by the Romans but, after their Empire crumbled, enjoyed little popularity until the thirteenth century, when public bathing came back in vogue for a while, reintroduced from the East by the returning Crusaders. It was not until the seventeenth century, however, that bathing became permanently re-established and even then it took over two hundred years to convince Europeans that it was a healthy, indeed necessary, procedure and should be performed regularly.

The seventeenth century also saw the introduction of 'sweating houses'. These were public 'Turkish' baths, a direct descendant of the Roman *caldarium* which the Turks had adopted and modified. They had become popular in Constantinople in the fifteenth century. Along with Turkish baths, scented baths were popular at this period. The great plague was still fresh in many memories, and people had begun to realise the importance of hygiene. At the same time perfumes were becoming more widely used. Their antiseptic value was more generally appreciated then than it is now, and a scented bath was both more enjoyable and more hygienic than an unscented one.

Nonetheless, Europeans were only slowly persuaded of the virtues of the bath. Without doubt people who inhabited warmer climates were better placed to appreciate them. They were also less likely to catch cold, which was the greatest fear of Europeans: at times bathing was regarded as a highly dangerous health risk, in which only foreigners or the foolhardy indulged. This attitude was slow to die out. Undoubtedly some unfortunate souls did succumb after braving the watery deeps; perhaps because their bodies were not used to it, and the water was too cold. As Daniel McKenzie writes:

> 'Our grandfathers ventured upon a bath only when it seemed to be called for — by others. Our grandmothers, with their clean, white cotton or linen undergarments had, or thought they had, even less need for it. Besides, in their prim and bashful eyes the necessary denudation antecedent to total immersion would have amounted, even when they were alone, to something like gross indecency. Before their time, again, in the eighteenth century, matters were even worse, for the society ladies of that day painted their faces *instead* of washing them, and mitigated the

effects of seldom-changed under-clothing by copiously drenching themselves with musk and other reliable perfumes.'

We still see many female faces which are never washed, but at least they are cleansed as well as painted!

Bathing did not become a widespread European habit until the nineteenth century. Even then it was at first done out of necessity, from a love of hygiene rather than a love of bathing. Daniel McKenzie comments:

> 'I can myself remember in my younger days in Scotland an old doctor having his first bath in the palatial surroundings of a modern bathroom. Not in his own house, needless to say! After a patient and particular inspection of all the glitting taps of "shower", "spray", "plunge", and what not, he commended his spirit to the Higher Powers. Then he proceeded gingerly to insert into the steaming water first of all his toes, then his feet, next his ankles, and so bit by bit, until, greatly daring, he had committed his entire body to the deep — to emerge as soon as possible!
> . . . His first bath! And his last! It nearly killed him, he said.'

It seems strange that the ancient Egyptians, Greeks, and Romans were enjoying the most luxurious baths several thousand years ago, while we in the West, particularly the English, have only recently 'taken the plunge'. The growth of the perfumed toiletries industry during the nineteenth and twentieth centuries has certainly helped to make bathing a more enjoyable pastime, although our modern, sophisticated perfumes are a far cry from the heavy, spicy, resinous perfumes of the ancient world.

Aromatic baths may affect us in a variety of ways. Firstly there is the fragrance of the essences used; if this is pleasing to the nose it will also please the spirit. Then there is the physiological action of the essence on the nervous system and the rest of the body, which takes place even though only a very small amount of the oil is absorbed through the skin.

A tepid bath ($28-35°C$) is relaxing and sedative. A hot bath ($35-39°C$) is tonifying if it is short, but if long is very debilitating. So a lavender bath, if the water is not too hot, will be relaxing, but a hot bath will tend to counteract the effect of lavender. Remember this when you take an aromatic bath, because many of the oils are either stimulating or relaxing. Most people prefer a stimulating bath in the morning, and a relaxing bath in the evening. But the best way to judge which essence to use is to use whatever you feel like at the time: your intuition knows what is good for you.

There are several ways you can use essences in the bath, and it is easy to make up a variety of bath oils. There are basically two types of bath oil: those which dissolve in the water, and those which do not. Taking the second type first, the most simple method is to scatter a few drops of pure essential oil into a full bath just before you get in. It is not a good idea to use any of these bath oils until the water has been run. If you do some of the essence will evaporate with the heat of the water before you even get into the bath. Any essential oil can be used in this way, but be careful not to use too much. Some essences are stronger than others, and some have a slightly irritating effect on the skin unless they are used very sparingly (e.g. basil, pepper, peppermint, rosemary); obviously this applies particularly to people with highly sensitive skins. If you are not sure, be cautious and use only two drops at first. If that amount does no harm you can increase it next time. On average, three to five drops is sufficient for most essences, although you may need up to ten or twelve for some. Experiment: you will soon find out what is best for you.

As soon as you have scattered the oil in the bath, swish the water gently so that the oil forms a film on top of it. (This is important, as sitting on a drop of neat essential oil can cause uncomfortable irritation!). This film will then envelop your skin. Now lie back and enjoy yourself! Do not expect to notice an immediate effect from the oils; they are very subtle, and their effect will be noticed later.

Another form of non-dissolving bath oil is a mixture of essential oil and vegetable oil. This is particularly useful if your skin tends to be dry. Any vegetable oil can be used, but avocado, sweet almond, and wheat germ oil are particularly nourishing because of their relatively high vitamin content. The amount of essence used is the same as for the above bath: anything between a half and three teaspoons of vegetable oil may be used. Mix the essence and fatty oil together, then add to the water in the same way as described for

for pure essence bath. Try mixing enough bath oil for several baths; if you feel adventurous you can mix several essences together. At first it is best to stick to one or two essences until you know which oils blend well, and in what proportions. Perfumery is an art, but it is surprising what can be done with a few essences and a little patience.

For the second type of bath oil — the one which dissolves in the water — you will need either shampoo, liquid soap, or washing-up detergent. Liquid soap and shampoo are both better for your skin than detergent. However, if you want a bubble bath detergent is the best thing to use — anything up to a tablespoon, depending on how many bubbles you want. Here again you can either add vegetable oil or not, but if you want a foam bath do not use it. If you do use oil a ratio of one part oil to three parts soap generally works well, but the proportion is flexible. Again experiment will show what suits you best. The amount of essence used is the same as described above.

Once in the bath the essences penetrate the skin in the same way as during an aromatherapy massage. This penetration is precipitated by the surrounding heat of the water. For the best therapeutic effect I would recommend using a non-soluble bath oil, so that the oil envelopes the body as you get in the water, and therefore stays next to the skin during the bath. Also a water-solubilised essence may not penetrate the skin so readily, since the skin does not absorb water. As you get out of the bath a small amount of oil will remain on your skin. If there is any oil still floating on the water it will cling to you as you emerge. Towel drying does not remove all of the essence and so the skin is left lightly perfumed.

You can reinforce your aromatic bath, especially if you have dry skin, by rubbing a scented oil over your body after drying. This protects the skin, keeps it healthy and supple, and gives you a faint, all-over fragrance. It also helps to counteract the drying effect of soap and water on the skin. You only need very little oil for this, and the best way to apply it is to cover both hands lightly with oil, and then rub it over your body.

Alternatively you could have someone else massage you after your bath. This is a very good time to have a massage, because your body is already relaxed and, to quote Dr William Martin Trinder (1812), 'After warm bathing, the application of an odoriferous oil on the skin is delightfully salubrious.' The

109

combination of bathing, massage, and aromatics must be one of the most relaxing luxuries in which one can indulge — and it is one that is good for you!

Public bathing (as opposed to swimming) has now been entirely replaced by bathing in the privacy of one's own home. Swimming baths do indeed have an aroma, and in that sense they are aromatic, but the smell of chlorine leaves much to be desired. The only form of public bathing nowadays which is cleansing is the steam or sauna baths. The sauna bath, which is almost a way of life in Finland, has enjoyed a growing popularity here in recent years. It is not practical, however, to use aromatics in combination with steam or sauna baths, since the main purpose of such baths is to induce elimination through the pores of the skin. The penetration of aromatic oils is therefore rendered impossible, or at least extremely difficult. However, after finishing a steam or sauna bath, when one is dry and has cooled down, massage may be given (one should wait at least half an hour, because the skin continues to perspire for some time after such baths). The combination of bath and massage is again very relaxing, and in this case perhaps even more 'salubrious'.

Here are some bath oil recipes which you can try for yourself, and a guide to help you make up your own recipes, with the approximate number of drops for use for each essence.

Winter bath — to help ward off colds, stimulate circulation

juniper	2 drops
lavender oil	3 drops

Summer bath — cooling, refreshing, invigorating

peppermint oil	1 drop
bergamot oil	4 drops

Morning bath — tonic, invigorating

rosemary oil	3 drops
juniper oil	2 drops

Evening bath — sedative, for those who have difficulty getting
to sleep

camomile oil	1 drop
lavender oil	4 drops

Aphrodisiac bath

ylang-ylang oil	1 drop
sandalwood oil	4 drops
jasmine oil (optional luxury!)	1 drop

Lemon bath — refreshing, relaxing, very cleansing

lemon juice from ½ lemon	
lemon oil	4 drops
geranium oil	1 drop

These recipes can be used either as they are, or with the addition of appropriate amounts of vegetable oil and/or soap. Quantities given are for one bath, although you may want to make up a larger quantity at a time.

Essences for baths — and how many drops to use

Relaxing		Tonic/stimulating	
Camomile	2	Basil	3
Cypress	4	Cardamom	3
Orange blossom	2	Peppermint	3
Lavender	4	Juniper	4
Marjoram	4	Hyssop	3
Rose	2	Rosemary	4
Sandalwood	4		
Clary sage	4		

Refreshing		Aphrodisiac	
Cypress	4	Jasmine	2
Lemon	4	Orange blossom	2
Peppermint	4	Rose	2
Basil	3	Sandalwood	4
Bergamot	4	Ylang-ylang	4
Geranium	4	Cardamom	3
Lavender	4		

If using more than one essential oil, keep the total number of drops to 5 or 6.

Therapeutic Baths

The history of the therapeutic use of water, both in the form of baths and otherwise, can be traced back as far as the ancient Egyptians. Since we can go this far back we may safely assume that water, being so integral a part of our lives, has been in therapeutic use ever since man realised that ill-health could be corrected and prevented. We may also hazard a guess that, since the Egyptians used both baths and aromatics so extensively, they may well have combined the two for therapeutic purposes.

We do know that Hippocrates, a Greek physician who lived c. 500 BC, considered water a serious therapeutic agent. Arabian physicians were using baths in the treatment of disease over a thousand years ago. First the Turks, then the French in the sixteenth century, and the English in the seventeenth adopted steam baths for pleasure, and also for therapy. In other parts of the world, such as America and Africa, the native tribes were using various forms of fumigations, hot-air baths, steam baths, and water baths, in the treatment of disease. In the nineteenth century various water cures were discovered, and became popular in Europe. Often they were effective in curing disease wihout any further treatment being given. Sebastian Kneipp, who is still remembered for his water treatments, cured the Archduke Joseph of Austria of Bright's disease in 1892.

In orthodox medical treatment the therapeutic use of water (hydrotherapy) is virtually obsolete. This is a pity, because cold water is an extremely good treatment for any kind of fever.

Water does not kill infection in such cases, but brings the temperature down very effectively, if correctly applied, giving much relief to the patient. The addition of a few drops of eucalyptus or peppermint oil to the water increases the effectiveness of this treatment. Cold compresses should be applied to the feet and forehead, the former being covered with a towel, and left until nearly dry. The hands may also be placed in bowls of cold water. In extreme cases the whole body should be wrapped in a cold, wet sheet. This should be soaked in water with eight drops of eucalyptus oil, and then firmly wrung before applying to the body. Then cover the patient with blankets and, if he feels very cold, tuck one or two hot water bottles in beside him. This type of treatment is far more effective, and far easier to apply, than the 'tepid sponging' used in hospitals. A constant watch should be kept on the temperature.

Water can be applied to the body in a variety of ways. As well as baths, steam baths, and compresses, there are sitz baths, hand baths, foot baths, douches, enemas, and sprays. There are also many types of bath employing other natural remedies, such as seaweed baths, brine baths, and so on. In each of these different types of application essential oils can be used, thereby giving a natural but considerable boost to the efficacy of the treatment. In most cases water itself is not sufficient to bring about a cure, nor is it intended to do so. But an aromatic water treatment is more powerful than hydrotherapy alone, and can often be an effective curative agent. In some cases it may be as effective as, or even more effective than, either aromatherapy massage or the internal use of oils. It therefore forms a very important part of aromatherapy.

The sitz bath consists of two sections: a large one, in which you sit, and a small one, for your feet. The water should come up to your waist, covering the lower abdomen. Because the two sections are separate the water in each can be kept at different temperatures. Sitz baths are generally used for diseases of the lower abdomen — urinary, genital, or intestinal disorders. They are especially useful for disorders of the uterus and female reproductive system. According to the problem being treated, appropriate essences may be added to the sitz bath. Leucorrhoea, amenorrhoea, dysmenorrhoea, and very occasionally even impotence (which is principally a psychological problem) may be treated in this way, and/or with a vaginal douche. The douche is necessary for leucorrhoea, and should be used daily. If you do not have a sitz bath a hip bath will do: run a bath so that the water comes up to the waist.

The same can be said of enemas, which may be given while fasting, or in constipation, diarrhoea, colitis, and other such disorders. Appropriate essences may be used to relax, tone up, de-toxify, or soothe the lower intestinal tract. Essential oils such as juniper or rosemary may be added to water sprays to increase the stimulating effect. These sprays are strong jets of water from a hose pipe, which are usually directed up and down the spine. They have a generally stimulating effect on the system, but are of particular use in spinal disorders, having the effect of deeply vibrating the joints, without any discomfort, and bringing considerable relief in chronic spinal conditions.

Hot, tepid, or cold compresses can be applied in a variety of disorders. They are commonly used for muscle spasm or bruising, but can be used, with essential oils diluted in water, for a variety of internal disorders. Compresses are made by mixing 2 drops of essential oil in 1 pint of warm water. (The same dilution or less should be used for hand, foot, and hip baths, and for douches and enemas.) Mix by shaking in a bottle, and soak a piece of material in the mixture. Anything that absorbs and is not too coarse will do, for example, a piece of old sheeting folded in four. Squeeze lightly , apply the compress to the skin, and cover with clothes and/or towelling. If the person needs to move about the compress can be bandaged in place. Leave for two to four hours or, if there is fever, until nearly dry; then replace the compress if necessary. An appropriate herbal infusion may be used instead of water.

Compresses should be applied over the affected area. If the kidneys are being treated, apply over the lower back; if the heart, apply to the chest, over the heart; if the intestines, apply to the abdomen, and so on. The effectiveness of these compresses has to be seen to be believed. Mességué once treated a man who could not urinate, and his doctors reckoned he had only a few hours to live. He applied a herbal compress to the man's back, over the kidney area. After about twenty minutes he began to urinate, and his life was undoubtedly saved. Aromatic compresses form a very useful home treatment, and can be applied daily by the patient in between visits to the therapist. Compresses may be left in place all night.

Foot and hand baths are used by Mességué in most of his treatments. As a home treatment they can be used instead of, or even in addition to, compresses. The water should be hot, but not unbearably so. The essences should be added just before immersing the hand or feet. Use about ten drops of essence for the foot bath. These baths should be used morning and evening, for not more than ten minutes, and should cover the ankles and wrists.

Hot-water foot baths used to be used as a treatment for colds, but now are only remembered by cartoonists. Sometimes powdered mustard (which is the most heating of all aromatics) was added to the bath in order to restore the natural heat of the body. Foot baths are very good for conditions of the head such as headache, migraine, colds, and facial neuralgia. They are also useful in disorders of the abdomen and legs, such as constipation, menstrual problems, and varicose veins. They are especially good for fatigue and congestive disorders. When taking a foot bath care should be taken to keep warm.

Aromatic waters are also useful for gargles in treating sore throats, mouth ulcers, and so on. Use 0.5% of essential oil in water. For sore throats also apply compresses to the upper neck. When preparing baths, douches, compresses, etc. always use warm to hot water unless there is a fever or great heat in part of the body, in which case cool to tepid water should be used.

Chapter 8

Massage

There are those who give with joy,
and that joy is their reward.
And there are those who give with pain,
and that pain is their baptism.
And there are those who give and know not
pain in giving, nor do they seek joy, nor
give with mindfulness of virtue;
They give as in yonder valley the myrtle
breathes its fragrance into space.
Through the hands of such as these God
speaks, and from behind their eyes he
smiles upon the earth.

The Prophet
Kahlil Gibran

Massage plays a very important role in aromatherapy. When using oils in aromatic massage, apart from the fact that the essences penetrate the skin, there is the added benefit of the massage itself, and also a psychological effect from the presence of the aroma. Massage is enjoyable to perform, and relaxing to receive; it is one of the best ways to relieve the stress and tension that most of us suffer from these days.

Massage is an ancient therapy. It is an extension of the instinctive urge to touch a painful part of the body, and often to rub it, as we do when bruised. The word 'anoint' is almost synonymous with massage, and the historic associations of the word show how old massage is. The ancients always used oils when giving a massage, and these were nearly always scented

116

oils. The earliest and principal form of aromatherapy is massage.

Massage also provides the means for patient-healer contact, which is a very important factor in healing, and is an easy and direct form of communication. Our hands are extremely sensitive, but as well as being tools for feeling, they are instruments of communication. The hand-healer communicates healing power through his hands, usually without even touching the body. We all have the ability to heal with our hands to some extent; massage and meditation are two ways of developing this. When we give a massage we communicate what we are feeling to the person we are massaging, so it is best to be in a calm, confident state of mind. Do not give a massage if you are feeling angry, tired, or nervous. It does not matter if your patient is not feeling good — your massage will help — provided you yourself are feeling confident and relaxed.

The first time that healer touches patient the hands should be receptive and reassuring. Before we can treat we need to know as much about the person as possible. While they are talking to us their body can be talking to our hands. The hands can tell us how much physical tension there is, and in which areas of the body; they help us to ascertain how receptive or nervous the patient is, the quality and texture of their skin, where there is muscle spasm, and perhaps why. The hands will discover congested areas, swollen parts, old sprains and strains. They will discover points which are sensitive, points which elicit pain somewhere else in the body. They may also tell us a great deal about the patient as a person.

When the hands have made their own 'diagnosis' they can begin to 'transmit' while still continuing to 'receive' if necessary. Our hands heal on two levels — the physical and what might be called the 'psychic'. Hand-healing has been called many things — faith healing, magnetic healing, spiritual healing, psychic healing, and so on. There is one thing we can be sure of, however: that some form of energy is transmitted from healer to patient through the hands. This has been known and used for thousands of years. Recently, the first scientific evidence to support this idea has come from Russia in the form of Kirlian photography.

Semyon Kirlian and his wife Valentina have discovered a method of photographing the aura of living plants and animals by placing them in a high-frequency electrical field. Photographs have shown that energy (exactly what this energy is has not been decided) shows up on photographs as luminescent clusters and flares. They are of different colours — blue, orange, yellow, violet — and are constantly moving, some quickly and some slowly. The Kirlians' experiments have shown that more light energy emits from the finger-tips than normal when a healer thinks about healing. That energy can be seen to come from the finger-tips is fascinating in itself. The fact that we may be able to control this energy in some way — and actually see the effects of this control as a change in light colour or intensity — is almost unbelievable. Only the most sceptical will refuse to believe that healing energy can be transferred from one person to another through the hands, but the possibility of scientific study of such phenomena has not until recently been seriously considered.

In order to heal you must be able to feel: to feel sympathy, compassion, and care for the other person. The more concentration and energy you put into your massage, the more easily that healing energy will be able to flow through you. The success of your massage depends not only on the type of massage you give, or how refined your technique is, as it does on your state of mind. If your mind is untroubled and you feel relaxed your movements will flow naturally.

Aromatherapy massage is a combination of swedish (soft-tissue) massage, shiatsu (acupuncture) massage, and neuro-muscular massage. Although these last two are virtually identical in technique they are based on different principles. In order to explain them clearly it is best to look at these three types of massage individually, and then see how they combine to form what we call aromatherapy massage.

Swedish Massage

Swedish massage is simply soft-tissue massage, or massage of the soft tissue of the body. It is so called because, early in the nineteenth century, a certain Professor Ling, who was Swedish, made a comprehensive scientific study of massage. He thus laid the foundations for what is now taught and practised as 'swedish massage'.

Swedish massage incorporates several different types of movement — stroking (effleurage), kneading, hacking, and cupping.

There is also petrissage, which is fairly deep massage with the thumbs; this is not much used in swedish massage, and will be discussed later. All the other movements are mostly superficial, and only affect the vascular and muscular system; all, that is, except for stroking which also has a reflex action on the nervous system. This is the type of movement we are primarily interested in, although kneading may occasionally be of use.

Effleurage

Stroking, or effleurage, is a slow, gentle, rhythmic movement of the whole hand, and is usually applied in an upward direction (i.e. towards the heart). The more pressure that is applied the deeper is the effect on the blood circulation and muscular tissue. The lighter it is (within certain limits) the greater is the reflex effect on the nervous system: this is particularly pleasant and relaxing.

The usual practice in swedish massage is to begin with effleurage. On the back (which is the area we are primarily concerned with) this is usually done by moving up the back, hands side by side, with the thumbs passing over the spine. Then the hands part outwards, over the shoulders, and move even more lightly down the sides of the back. There are several variations of this, but I have found this to be the most generally useful method. One variation which is sometimes useful is to stand at the patient's head, and to perform the same movement in reverse, going down the spine and then up the sides of the back. Stroking is used in a similar manner on the rest of the body. On the leg, for instance, with the patient lying prone (face down), massage from just above the heel to the top of the leg; the hands are kept parallel and just touching on the way up, and separate at the top, coming down the sides of the leg.

In this movement there is a slight pressure on the upward stroke, and no pressure at all on the downward stroke. The pressure on the upward stroke can be varied according to need, but it is generally best to start with a very light pressure, gradually becoming heavier. More pressure will be needed on heavily built people, and less on frailer physiques. Do not use much pressure on very nervous people. When doing effleurage the hands should be neither tense nor floppy, but firm and flexible so they adapt and mould to the contours of the body as they pass over the skin. Usually the fingers are held together, but they may be spread if you like, especially when doing effleurage with only one hand. This is sometimes necessary, as when massaging the arm, where there is not enough room for two hands together. Effleurage can be done over any part of the body, whether bony or muscular.

Kneading

This movement is not used as much in aromatherapy as in swedish massage, of which it is an essential part. Kneading is done with the whole hand, or hands, and is basically a squeezing and rolling movement. In order to 'squeeze' and 'roll' you have first to 'pick up', and kneading is easiest to do on the more fleshy parts of the body. It cannot be done on the more bony parts, such as hands, wrists, elbows, etc. Pick up the part being massaged with the two thumbs 'opposing' the other four fingers. Then lift, squeezing just enough to keep hold of the muscle, and roll, so that the hand slides across the surface of the skin. The hands can then either return to their original position by lightly passing back over the same area (as in the return movement of effleurage) or they can 'knead' their way back again, doing the same movement but in reverse. A further variation is to have one hand 'kneading' towards you while the other hand 'kneads' away from you. This is a little more difficult but is very beneficial if you can master it. This movement can only be done on the most fleshy parts, while one-handed kneading is easier on the less fleshy ones. When kneading be careful not to pinch or to squeeze too hard; it is as much a rolling movement as a squeezing one.

Kneading is useful for aching muscles — aching calves after a long walk, aching back after gardening — or tense muscles, especially that part of the trapezius muscle between neck and shoulders. Muscles begin to ache when the chemical by-products of 'muscle combustion' (mainly lactic acid) begin to build up in the tissues. This usually happens when muscles are being used beyond their normal capacity, and the blood and lymph cannot eliminate the lactic acid quickly enough from the area. Massage, especially kneading, stimulates the circulation and helps to disperse lactic acid deposits.

Swedish massage is easy to do. Even if you massage fairly heavily you should not hurt anybody, but it is best to be gentle, flowing, and sensitive. Once you have mastered the basic techniques you can improvise your own strokes: you will probably find this happening quite naturally. Because it is easiest to do, and the least potentially harmful, you should learn swedish massage before attempting to do any deep massage. You should also have a reasonable knowledge of anatomy so that you know what you are massaging; and of physiology to help you understand why you are massaging.

Neuromuscular Massage

Neuromusuclar means nerve-muscle. This is a type of massage which has been developed by Western osteopaths and masseurs, mostly in the USA. Basically it is a form of deep massage which is intended to reach nerves, ligaments, tendons, and other connective tissue not normally reached by soft-tissue massage. Neuromuscular massage does not normally come within the scope of aromatherapy massage, but I have included a description of it here as it is very useful, and its practice at present is not widely known.

Like most methods of deep massage, neuromuscular massage is performed with the pads of the thumbs and/or fingers. A certain amount of pressure is required — as a general rule not more than 5 kg, although 15 kg or more may occasionally be used by experienced masseurs. (The pressure exerted may be tested out by pressing with thumb or finger on your bathroom scales.) Several movements are used, the most usual being a circular movement. The thumb or finger is placed on the skin, and then performs small circles, moving over the underlying tissues but keeping contact with the same area of skin. This is very good for medium-depth massage, and useful when giving a general massage or when very deep massage is not desirable. For deeper penetration a sawing type of movement is used. While pressure is maintained, move the thumb or finger backwards and forwards along the same line, again keeping contact with the same area of skin. 'Sawing' is a very deep movement, and is often painful, although this also depends on the amount of pressure exerted. Do not use it for more than twenty seconds on the same area, or for more than a total of ten minutes in one massage session. It can also cause slight bruising. This is sometimes inevitable, and some people bruise very easily, but it should be avoided where possible.

The third movement is not really a movement, merely a downward pressure. It is almost as deep as sawing, but not so painful,

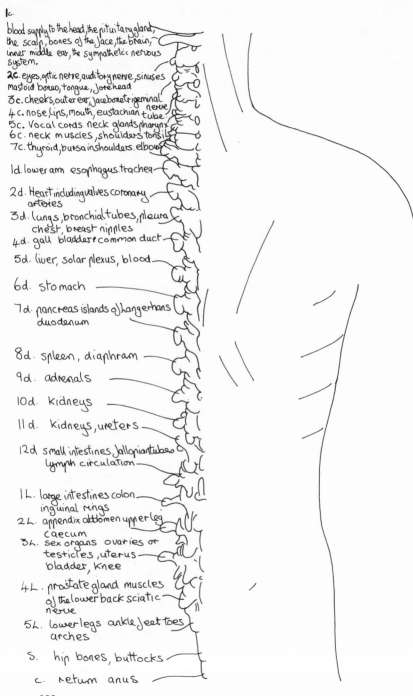

1c.
blood supply to the head, the pituitary gland, the scalp, bones of the face, the brain, inner middle ear, the sympathetic nervous system.

2c. eyes, optic nerve, auditory nerve, sinuses mastoid bones, tongue, forehead

3c. cheeks, outer ear, facebone trigeminal nerve

4c. nose, lips, mouth, eustachian tube.

5c. Vocal cords neck glands pharynx

6c. neck muscles, shoulders tonsils

7c. thyroid, bursa in shoulders. elbows

1d. lower arm esophagus. trachea

2d. Heart including valves coronary arteries

3d. lungs, bronchial tubes, pleura chest, breast nipples

4d. gall bladder & common duct

5d. liver, solar plexus, blood

6d. stomach

7d. pancreas islands of hangerhans duodenum

8d. spleen, diaphram

9d. adrenals

10d. kidneys

11d. kidneys, ureters

12d small intestines fallopian tubes lymph circulation

1L. large intestines colon inguinal rings

2L. appendix abdomen upper leg caecum

3L. sex organs ovaries or testicles, uterus bladder, knee

4L. prostate gland muscles of the lower back sciatic nerve

5L. lower legs ankle feet toes arches

S. hip bones, buttocks

c. retum anus

and can be used more freely. As in the other movements the amount of pressure should be geared to the pain response: a certain amount of discomfort is expected, but never intense pain. When doing any form of massage which requires pressure it is usually easier to use the thumbs, since they are stronger than the fingers, and can withstand more pressure for a longer time. On the other hand you may find it less of a strain to alternate between thumbs and fingers. It is also much easier to use your body-weight — by keeping your arm straight, and leaning over the patient — than it is to apply pressure using your hand and arm muscles alone. This may feel strange at first, but in the end is much less tiring.

By massaging the area immediately to either side of the spine one can give a massage which is stimulating and relaxing at the same time. The result is that the patient feels much more relaxed, while at the same time his whole body, including the internal organs, has been toned up. This happens because the nerves which are massaged constitute the nerve supply to the whole body (except for the head which is suppled by the cranial nerves). This does not mean that spinal massage makes further massage unnecessary, but it does make the spine the most important area in the body for deep massage.

There are two ways in which you can use the diagram of spinal nerve roots. Firstly if you know that a certain area or organ needs treating, you should devote more time to massaging the corresponding spinal nerves. By doing this you stimulate the nerve supply to that area, which then receives more energy, thus stimulating cell renewal, relieving congestion, and so on. If you find the spinal area painful you can be sure it needs massage. Secondly, by massaging the whole spinal area, you will find certain spots which are particularly painful. These areas need special attention, and care for deep massage: they may also — though not necessarily — indicate trouble in the organs supplied by those nerves. The area we are concerned with lies between the spine, and the ridge of muscle lying an inch or so to the side of it. This 'gutter' is, very conveniently, just wide enough for the thumb. You can use any of the three movements described above — circling, sawing, or pressing — and work on both sides of the spine at once, or do them one at a time, working upwards or downwards as you prefer.

Neuromuscular massage is very useful for sprained joints, strained muscles, muscular tension, or spasm, and sundry related problems. It can also be used to stimulate nerves as described above, and so may lend itself to a wide variety of complaints as an auxiliary therapy. Much of this type of massage is done on the origins and insertions of muscles. It is interesting to note that these points sometimes correspond exactly with acupuncture points. All muscles, except for a few on the face, are attached to bone at either end. The attachment takes the form of a bundle of white tissue which we call a tendon. Some tendons are extremely short, while some are several inches long. The points of attachment are called the origins and insertions. The origin is the more fixed point, and the insertion is on the bone which the muscle moves. The origin of the calf muscle, for example, is at the knee, while the insertion is at the heel; the origin of the biceps is at the shoulder, and the insertion is at the elbow.

Massage on the origins and insertions (O. and I. massage) has a stimulating (yang) effect. If a muscle is atonic (too relaxed, too yin) O. and I. massage will have a tonic effect, and so help to restore normality. This type of massage also helps to prevent the wasting of muscles; it stimulates cell regeneration, and helps to keep the blood and nerve supplies to the muscle healthy. If you want to know what neuromuscular massage feels like try massaging the area where the back of the neck meets the skull, getting your thumbs under the ridge of bone you will feel there. This area is painful in most people, especially towards the outside. Use enough pressure to make it hurt, though not unbearably. As well as massaging the insertions of twelve muscles you are massaging seven acupuncture points. Massage of this area helps to relax the head and neck, and is very good for headaches, which are often related to congestion and tenstion at the back of the neck.

If a muscle is too tense (too yang) O. and I. massage does not increase the muscle tension, and may even help to normalise the condition. There is also a method for treating muscle spasm, which is to press on the centre or belly of the muscle. The result is an expansive, relaxing, yin effect. Pressure should be exerted for about one minute, without any movement. Make sure you are on the centre of the muscle. Most people's spines need neuromuscular massage. Because we wear shoes, walk on concrete, sit badly, and so on, our backs usually suffer in time. Bone manipulation may be necessary, but in the majority of cases several treatments of neuromuscular massage are sufficient to correct any problem which is not serious. On the other hand manipulation which is performed without also giving deep massage often fails to correct the problem, which involves ligaments and muscles as much as bones. The result is that an endless series of manipulations are given, with only a slight improvement to show for it. On most backs you will find small knots of tension — muscle spasm — next to the spine. Sometimes they are so obvious you can see them quite clearly. These are the spots that need pressure, and they are always painful. Quite often you will hear a small click as the bone readjusts itself without any forceful manipulation being used.

Neuromuscular massage is not something you should attempt without some form of training in massage. It requires the exertion of quite heavy pressure and you might hurt someone through lack of practical knowledge.

Shiatsu Massage

The word shiatsu comes from the Japanese *shi*, finger, and *atsu*, pressure. Like acupuncture and moxibustion, it is a branch of oriental medicine. All these processes work on the principles of *Chi* and yin/yang, and treatment is applied by affecting the energy flow of the meridians. The points used vary considerably from one person to another, since the approach is highly individual and not symptomatic. The number of points used also varies, but is usually between five and ten. Shiatsu is not so concerned with exact, individual points. Indeed those of us who are not trained acupuncturists would not be capable of giving such specialist treatment.

Shiatsu massage is fairly vigorous and, like neuromuscular massage, can be painful and cause mild bruising. Although it is occasionally necessary to massage deeply on painful spots it is important not to cause a great deal of pain. The level of pain should be kept below that which is comfortable to the patient and pressure on painful spots should constitute less than 10% of the total time given to massage. It is usually the case that an area or point which is painful to the touch needs to be massaged. These spots are not painful until they are pressed, and after massage the pain is subdued or completely gone. This applies both to shiatsu and neuromuscular massage.

Generally speaking shiatsu is performed by massaging along the meridians. In a whole body massage one starts at the head, working down the back, then from the hands up to the shoulders, and from the feet up to the pelvis; all the time following the tracts of meridians. When doing the arms, for instance, several journeys are necessary in order to follow all the meridians in the arm. The actual method of pressure is similar to that used in neuromuscular massage, and is not as important as the fact of pressure being applied to the correst area. There are two ways of pressing: either simple pressure or pressure with a small circular movement. The thumbs are most often used. Pressure is applied about every inch along each meridian. In shiatsu it is not important to press very deeply, since one is not trying to massage nerves or ligaments which lie deep in the tissues. Shiatsu is more like an energy massage — application of *Ch'i*, or vital force, rather than physical force.

In order to give Ch'i, or energy, in massage it is necessary to understand certain points. The masseur must be in a reasonably good state of health, otherwise he will only deplete his already depleted Ch'i; he should at least be stronger in this sense than the person he is massaging. Some people may feel that they do not give their own energy in massage or healing, but are merely channels through which energy, perhaps divine energy, flows; they do not consider therefore that they deplete their own energy. The individual attitude is all-important here: if you feel your source of energy is the Divine Will or the Cosmic Energy Force you will be able to heal by this means. Conversely if you feel that massage is going to deplete your own energy, then it probably will do so. When you are giving the massage (and also prior to giving it) you should be in a peaceful state of mind, a state of non-thinking. Meditation is the only way to accomplish this. If you have no knowledge of meditation you should concentrate all your attention on the massage itself. Breathe slowly and deeply into the abdomen keeping it, and the rest of your body, as relaxed as possible. Encourage the patient also to take a few deep breaths if he does not naturally do this (which he should if you are sufficiently relaxed and open yourself). By concentrating on one point you will find it easier to relax, and your massage will be more relaxing, and less draining on you. If you do happen to be in an anxious state of mind this simple form of meditation, plus the aroma of the essences you are using, will make you, as well as the patient, feel better. Also, by concentrating on your hands and the massage they are giving, you are encouraging subtle energy to flow through them. Do not just go through the motions of massaging while your mind is on something completely different. 'Feel the essence' of your actions; concentrate on what you are doing.

Shiatsu has two purposes. One is to charge the patient's Ch'i generally, the other is to massage certain meridians and specific points. Again we find that the back is the most important area for massage. The bladder meridian has two tracts on either side of the spine. Each of these tracts has a number of points which relate to all the other meridians (and hence organs) in the body. One tract (which we can call tract A) runs about three-quarters of an inch to the side of spine. The other (tract B) runs about an inch farther out from tract A, and follows a line down from the inner corner of the shoulder blade.

There is also a meridian — the governing vessel — which runs up the very centre of the back and head. The energy flow of the bladder meridian goes from head to foot. Massage with this flow, in a downward direction, will give a generally stimulating effect; massage against the flow, upwards, will have a more relaxing effect. Massage of these two meridians forms an important part of aromatherapy massage.

Aromatherapy Massage

> '*Non-interrupting* attitude of mind constitutes the most vital element in the art of fencing as well as in Zen. If there is space for even the breadth of a hair between two actions, this is interruption. For example, when the hands are clapped, the sound issues without a moment's deliberation. Likewise one movement must follow another without being interrupted by one's conscious mind.'

So Glen Barclay writes in *Mind over Matter*. Non-interrupting attitude of mind is his term for meditation, a state of mind also of great importance in massage, where a continual flow of movement is desirable. Although aromatherapy massage incorporates the deep thumb pressures of shiatsu and neuromuscular massage as well as the soothing effleurage of swedish massage the total effect should be harmonious, and not jar in any way. Deep massage should be done gently rather than vigorously; in this way pressure can be applied which is effective and at the same time causes the minimum of discomfort. For this reason I do not advocate the use of hacking, cupping, or the more vigorous, sudden movements associated with shiatsu. Neither would I recommend the use of the deep sawing movement used in neuromuscular massage. Although this is effective for massaging ligaments and nerves it is painful and not really necessary in aromatherapy.

We are now left with two movements: the effleurage of swedish massage and the deep thumb pressure of shiatsu and neuromuscular massage. This can be applied in three ways: either by pressure with no movement, pressure with small circular movements, or by a movement we have not discussed so far. This is the application of pressure while sliding the thumb along a certain path, whether it be a meridian, nerve tract, or muscle. This last movement is particularly useful as it is fairly deep, the action is smooth, and every inch of the meridian or nerve tract is covered. It is a sliding movement, and can only be used in an oil massage. There are other movements which may be occasionally used for one reason or another, and every masseur has his own preferences, and improvises his own movements. The ones I recommend seem to me to be the most generally useful for our purposes, and would certainly provide the basis for any good aromatherapy massage.

Before going any further with the massage itself let us take a look at the purposes of aromatherapy massage. It aims:

> to aid oil penetration
>
> to stimulate generally and/or relax
>
> to treat locally
>
> to treat via nerve supply, reflexes, or meridians.

We might also add that it is intended to guide the essences to those areas where they are most needed.

For effective skin penetration of the oils the skin must be able to receive them; it must not be congested, either from the inside with toxins or from the outside with dirt. The condition of the skin is partly affected by the condition of the blood, which itself needs to be 'clean' in order to carry the oils through the body. The lymph, even more than the blood, will not carry the oils efficiently if it is already congested. Lymph does not have a pump like the heart, and relies on muscle movements and gravity for its flow. Thus, when congested, it tends to stagnate. Lymph stagnation is associated with oedema, aching muscles, obesity, cellulitis, swollen glands, and so on. The causes of blood toxicity, lymph stagnation, and the resulting skin congestion are usually lack of exercise, overeating, poor diet (too many unnatural foods, etc.), and most commonly, constipation; in some cases congestion may also be the result of functional disturbances.

Since skin congestion is a considerable barrier to aromatherapy massage, its cause must be corrected before any successful treatment can be given. All of the conditions mentioned in connection with lymph stagnation, plus tiredness, sallow complexion, boils, acne, and often oily skin, are signs of congestion. In some cases a short fast followed by an improvement in the diet will be sufficient to relieve the congestion. In other cases more extensive treatment will be necessary. This is not to say that aromatherapy treatment cannot be given to people with congested skin — in fact it can often help to treat congestion — but additional means should be employed whenever it is necessary.

For maximum receptivity the pores (hair follicles) of the skin should be wide open and peripheral blood circulation should be full. This state can be achieved by applying radiant heat to the skin, and/or by friction massage, which is performed by rubbing the hand to and fro across the skin fairly quickly. This should be done before any oil is applied and will cause a mild hyperaemia, redness due to the capillaries swelling with blood. Radiant heat lamps are not always available, so let me emphasise that you do not have to use heat. Friction massage is at least as good, and is usually quicker.

Stimulating	Relaxing
More deep, strong movements	More gentle, superficial movements
Massaging down the bladder meridian and up the governor	Flow of movement should never be broken
	Massaging up the bladder meridian and down the governor

This table is of course relative: any massage is both stimulating and relaxing. The terms may indeed be confusing, the same massage or essence being both stimulating and relaxing: stimulating to one system and relaxing to another, or stimulating when energy is lacking, and relaxing when energy is in excess. The aim of both the table and the massage is to create a balance, to restore harmony between the different parts and functions of the body.

If there is a local problem — an aching shoulder, oedematic ankles, or the like — the massage will be specifically aimed at treating the problem. This may involve a great deal of effleurage around the area, the stimulation of local nerve supply, and massaging local meridians and acupuncture points. If there is an organic malfunction — a tired heart, poor digestion, etc. — specific treatment will also be given both locally, as described above, and sometimes on distant meridians or reflexes which relate to the problem. If there is no apparent problem a general, full body massage may be given. Aromatherapy massage can take three forms: back massage, facial massage, and whole body massage. When giving a whole body massage it is best to start with the back, so that your patient is already well relaxed when you go on to attend the rest of the body.

Back Massage

Before applying any oil give a fairly vigorous friction massage to the whole area, using the palms of your hands. This should take less than a minute; now apply the oil. Always pour into your hand, not directly on to your patient. Only use as much as you need; you can apply more oil later on if necessary. Now gently effleurage the whole area, as described in the section on swedish massage, for about one minute. Now gently knead the neck and shoulders for about thirty seconds each. (It is very important, when doing back massage, to work along the whole area of the spine from the coccyx to the base of the skull.) Now, using the thumbs, one behind the other, slide (with pressure) up the spine itself, from one end to the other. Be careful not to press too hard when you come to the neck area. Repeat once. Now do the same movement along the area immediately to either side of the spine (nerve roots and bladder meridian tract A). You can do both sides at once, or one at a time. If your hands are weak, and you cannot get sufficient pressure, you can use the outer edge of one thumb, and press on top of it with the heel of your other hand. The fingers on both hands should be completely relaxed. Now repeat the movement, this time along bladder meridian tract B on both sides. These last two movements should take about thirty seconds each. You have now completed the basic unit of an aromatherapy back massage which should take about three minutes. It is important to complete this unit in three or four minutes, because of the continual evaporation of essences.

Now we repeat this same basic movement, this time taking longer and concentrating more on specific area. Repeat the friction, especially over the spinal area, then the effleurage again over the whole back, then the kneading, this time covering a larger area, and going a little deeper. You should give the neck plenty of kneading, and cover also the whole shoulder area, and the waist-hip area. Repeat the sliding pressure on the spine, nerve roots, and bladder meridian, but this time concentrate more on painful areas, or areas which you know need stimulation. Also massage any other points on the back which you know need massage. These may include acupuncture points, neuromuscular points, reflex points, etc. Do not use maximum pressure this time, and do not spend too long on a single point.

Now we come to the third and final stage which is basically another repetition, but this time leave out the friction and concentrate even more on points or areas which need attention, giving them more time and more pressure. Finish with effleurage, at first fairly deep then getting progressively lighter. Your back massage is now complete. I have purposely been very precise here to give you a clear idea of what is required, but inevitably there are many variations and alternatives. Once you have mastered the basic techniques you can improvise around that structure. The times given are also approximate, and will inevitably vary from masseur to masseur and from patient to patient.

Whole Body Massage

Head

Here we begin with head massage, in which no oil is used (you could use oil on a bald head). Head massage can also be given as a preliminary to a back massage. First effleurage the whole head (except for the face), using both hands at once and moving from front to back. You can alternate these straight movements with circular movements. If you do this both hands should describe the circles in unison; not alternately. Then friction using the fingertips, as if you were shampooing, again moving from front to back. You will need to do four or five movements to cover the

131

whole area. Now, using either simple pressure or small circular movements, massage along the governor meridian (centre of the head) from the bridge of the nose to the nape of the neck, then the bladder meridian, and the gall bladder. Each meridian should be massaged three times from front to back. Finish with light effleurage.

Back

Follow the same procedure as described above.

Chest

Using ony three fingers of each hand to begin this massage, start under the chin, with finger-tips facing each other (elbows out). Gently stroke down the throat to the foot of the sternum (breast bone), gradually turning in the hands till they are pointing downwards.

In a continuous movement, return the hands to level above the breast, revolving them until the finger-tips are facing each other again. Now, with a slight pause and hands slightly cupped, press gently over the area above the breasts. Continue in an outward and upward movement towards the shoulders, with hands revolving till finger-tips are pointing downwards. With the outside edge of the hands (little finger) press quite firmly into the area between the body and the top of the arm (axilla). Then, still using the whole of the hand, make a firm return movement across the back of the shoulders to the base of the neck.

Without stopping, and now only using three fingers, return to a lighter movement, and move forward under the jaw line to the starting-point under the chin. Repeat the entire procedure. The only slight pressures used in this massage are over the lymphatic glands.

Abdomen

The abdomen is a very responsive area for it is here that we can apply massage to some of the internal organs; it is also a common seat of tension and fear. It is especially important when massaging the abdomen not to use too much pressure. With experience you will become sensitive to each patient, and you will know how hard to press on which areas. In the meantime do not be afraid — but be gentle. Begin with light friction, then apply oil and begin effleurage. I find this easiest to do with one hand performing a circle round the navel. Do plenty of effleurage on the abdomen. Start lightly, gradually applying more pressure, but never enough to cause discomfort. The next movement consists of pressure with circular movements along the colon. Start at point A (the caecum), then massage up the ascending colon to point B (the hepatic flexure). This should be given extra massage, especially if it is tender. Then massage along the transverse colon to point C (the splenic flexure) which also needs special attention, then down the descending colon, finishing at point D. Now repeat the whole movement, concentrating more on any points which are tender, but be very gentle: the abdomen is a sensitive area, and should always be treated with the utmost care. Next we go from a point just below the navel (E) up to the point of the breast bone (F). The starting-point is actually the second chakra and point F

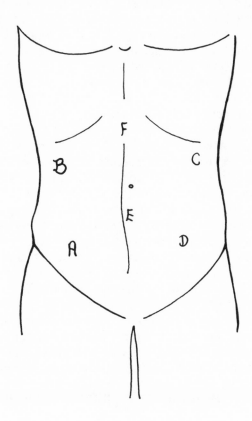

is the third chakra, or solar plexus. The massage here can consist of either circular movements or pressure. The third and final part involves massaging the lower ege of the liver and the spleen. Massage from just above point B, to the solar plexus (F), and then to just above point C. Again you can use either pressure or circular movements. Finish with plenty of effleurage. By covering the areas described here you are also massaging several important acupuncture points on different meridians.

Arms and legs

In a whole body massage we cannot leave out the limbs, although they are not of great importance in aromatherapy as far as oil penetration is concerned. There are many important acupuncture points in the lower half of each limb; in fact acupuncture treatment can be given only using points located in these area. They are particularly sensitive because it is here that yang energy turns into yin energy, and vice versa. For leg and arm massage use the same formula: friction, effleurage, kneading (optional), and deep pressure. You should massage up the limb, especially on the legs. Never press into the area at the back of the knee. Do not forget the hands and feet; they are sensitive areas, and like being massaged. If you want to follow the exact meridian tracts get a good book on acupuncture and study them.

The essential in all aromatherapy massage is to keep it smooth and flowing. Sometimes, after you have been massaging for two or three minutes, red lines or patches appear on the back, which stay for one or two minutes and then disappear. If you are fairly quick you can massage where the lines appear before they disappear again. These are particular spots which need pressure, and the body is telling you exactly where to press. You will invariably find that they are sore spots: they may be areas of congestion, acupuncture points, or meridians. I have seen this phenomenon on a number of backs, and it seems to occur more readily when essences are being used in the massage. When it happens you can be sure you are giving a really good treatment.

There are certain parts of our body which our worries, fears, and inhibitions keep in an almost permanent state of tension. Areas commonly affected are the jaws, neck and shoulders, abdomen, and buttocks. Although massage cannot, in itself, remove the fear or whatever is causing the tension, it is surprising how much it can accomplish in combination with an understanding attitude and sympathetic ear. Sometimes, if you hit on one of these cores of tension the patient will start to unburden himself of his troubles.

A great deal obviously depends on the relationship between therapist and patient. It is important for the patient to relax and to feel at ease. Talking, or even crying, is sometimes necessary for him to release this tension. Although massage will help some, it will not accomplish very much if the patient fights it. Sometimes however the patient will simple feel enormously relaxed and relieved, although not manifesting this in any obvious way such as crying. We all have areas of tension, and massaging them always helps, whether or not it produces a dramatic release of tension.

The jaws can be massaged during either head or facial massage. The points to concentrate on are: about one inch above the angle of the jaw, and the temples. Quite often the muscles around the hip bone also need attention. You need quite a bit of pressure on the buttocks to get through to the deeper muscles. The neck and shoulders can be done during either head or back massage. We have already mentioned the points at the base of the occiput. Also press deeply on either side of the cervical spine (pressing inwards and forwards) and outwards from the base of the neck (pressing downwards). Here you are also following the tracks of the small and large intestine meridians.

Remember, massage is mantric; it is something which can take you and the patient out of yourselves for a time. This is a secret of a good relaxing massage. Keep it rhythmical and flowing, get the patient to breathe deeply and relax, and if necessary tell him to close his eyes and concentrate on your hands, that is on the massage itself. If patients lie there thinking away at their usual pace — and the chances are they are worrying about something — they will not get anything like the full benefit of a good massage.

Reflexology

This is not just another type of massage, it is an exact and useful method of diagnosis and treatment, and is a valuable adjunct to aromatherapy massage. Reflexology was brought from the East by an American, Dr Fitzgerald. Although there are some parallels between it and acupuncture, it is a different method based on different principles. Fitzgerald treated patients using reflexes all over the body, but for the sake of clarity and simplicity we need only consider those on the feet. These are the most generally useful reflexes, and possibly the most sensitive.

Reflexology (or zone therapy) is based on the principle that the body can be divided into ten zones, five on each side of a central, vertical line. All organs which are situated in the middle — such as the bladder, thyroid, and stomach — are found in the first zone on both feet. If there is trouble in an organ, other organs in the same zone may be affected. An organ on the left side of the body — such as the spleen — is only found on the left foot, and the same applies to the right side of the body. As you can see in the diagram all the organs are logically placed with the eyes, ears, sinuses, etc. around the toes, the kidneys about half-way down the foot and so on.

The type of massage used in reflexology is rather different from that used in neuromuscular or shiatsu massage. The side of the thumb farthest away from the fingers is used, in small, circular movements. There is a simple rule of thumb in reflexology: if it hurts, massage it. It is, however, important to realise that you are exiting a reflex pain, and not an ordinary foot pain. A reflex pain feels exactly as if you are massaging the foot with your finger-nail (which you should never do), or as if something sharp is being driven into the foot. Quite often the patient will jump, and hastily draw his foot away.

Reflexology is a valuable aid to diagnosis. If someone has a pain in a certain area of the body you can often find out which organ is responsible for the pain by this type of foot massage. By massaging the whole reflex area in both feet you can tell which parts are not functioning correctly at that time, and also treat the affected parts in the same way, by reflex massage. Although this is a simple and harmless method of treatment it can often produce surprising results. As in any type of massage it is important not to hurt the patient unduly, and not to give too much treatment to one spot.

Solar Plexus
This reflex is often sore when the patient suffers from nervous tension or other nervous complaints.

Large Intestine
Reflex massage often helps considerably in cases of constipation, one of the commonest modern complaints.

Prostate
Massage of this reflex will help in all kinds of prostate disorders.

Ovaries
All kinds of female complaints may be helped by massaging the reflex to the ovaries; also check the uterus and fallopian tube reflexes for tenderness. Also massage the pituitary and thyroid relfexes if tender.

Pituitary
This is the master gland, and should never be omitted when checking the reflexes. Massage of the pituitary reflex will usually benefit disorders which involve any of the other endocrine glands.

Sinuses
Massaging these reflexes will help to relieve catarrhal congestion, colds, etc.

Cellulitis
Massage the lymphatic zones for cellulitis, fluid retension, obesity.

Menopause
Work on the glands and the solar plexus.

Asthma
Work on the endocrine glands, especially the adrenals, and also the lungs and lymphatics.

Varicose Veins
Work on the large intestine, and check the small intestine, liver, kidneys, and lungs.

Congestion
In any condition that involves congestion check the eliminative organs: large intestine, kidneys, lungs, and also the liver and lymphatics.

Congestion can take many forms: catarrh, constipation, varicose veins, cellulitis, tiredness, depression, and so on. It cannot be cured by reflexology or aromatheraphy unless the underlying cause is sought out and corrected. This may be psychological — congestion can be caused by mental tension creating physical

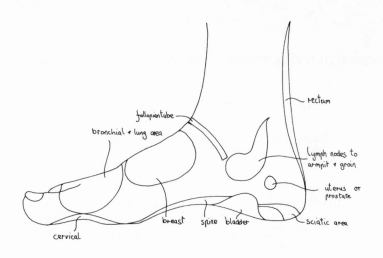

rectum

fallopian tube

bronchial & lung area

lymph nodes to
armpit & groin

uterus or
prostate

cervical

breast   spine bladder

sciatic area

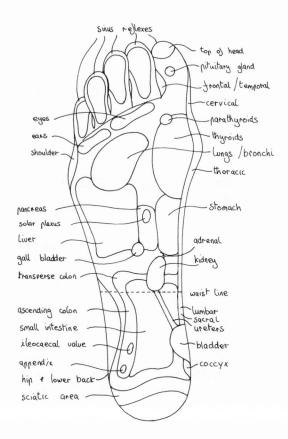

sinus reflexes

top of head

pituitary gland

frontal / temporal

cervical

parathyroids

eyes

thyroids

ears

lungs / bronchi

shoulder

thoracic

pancreas

stomach

solar plexus

liver

adrenal

gall bladder

kidney

transverse colon

waist line

ascending colon

lumbar
sacral
ureters

small intestine

ileocaecal valve

bladder

appendix

coccyx

hip & lower back

sciatic area

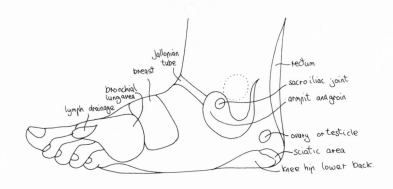

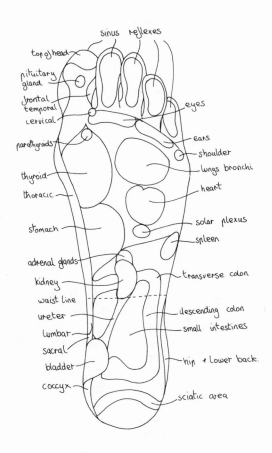

tension — or purely physical — faulty diet, lack of exercise, over-eating; usually more than one factor is involved.

Facial Massage

A good facial massage with essential oils is a delightful and uplifting experience. From the time the hands start to apply the oil, it is one continuous rhythmic movement. There are no heavy movements at all.

The best treatment is given when the patient is reclining in a completely relaxed position, with the neck and shoulders free of clothing. The neck at least must be free, as no facial massage should be given without treating the neck.

With the hair free of the face, and the neck free of the couch, the skin is gently cleansed and tissue dried. The appropriate aromatic facial oil is chosen: a light vegetable oil with the pure essences appropriate to the skin to be treated, or a ready made-up aromatic facial oil. Sufficient oil should be taken to cover the face and neck. Usually about half a teaspoonful (2½ ml) is sufficient, although some particularly absorbent skins will require more.

Start with both hands under the chin, finger-tips touching, fingers closed. Wrists must be supple and hands pliable and moulding.

Work out towards the ear and return hands to centre. Then with the whole hand, smooth across the face to the temple. Turning wrists in towards you, travel gently with the fingers under the eyes, up the bridge of the nose to the forehead, then over the eyebrows and gently back under the eyes again, and up from the nose-bridge over the forehead to the hair line. Continue with palming movements on the forehead. These soothing movements from nose-bridge to hair line are used several times between other movements. Then stroke down the nose, chin, and throat in one continuous line and oil the neck.

Without pausing, return to the original position and repeat the massage, remembering that movements should go across lines. Work on the main area of the face with the whole hand to begin with, going from chin to temple. Work round the eyes, using only one finger of each hand. Proceed from the temples, under the eyes and up the forehead to the hair line. Incorporate movements to suit the type of skin, ensuring that the procedure is flowing.

After finishing the neck, give a complete effleurage on face and neck, becoming lighter and lighter, and finish with a light palming on the forehead, and vibration over the eyes.

Hints on Massage

The massage room should be well-lit, but without glaring lights. Especially when doing oil massage the room must be warm enough for the patient. Cover up with a towel any parts not actually being massaged. If they are still partly clad, protect clothing with paper towelling; oil can be very messy if it gets on your clothes.

Make sure that your patient is comfortable and warm before you begin.

Always wash your hands before and after giving a massage. Remember to replace the cap on your bottle of oil, to prevent the evaporation of the essences. It is very difficult to do massage on the floor, because the masseur has to keep moving about; it is not only tiring, but makes some movements difficult to perform. Most couches for swedish massage are about 2 ft 6 in. high. For aromatherapy I would recommend something slightly lower, between 2 ft and 2 ft 2 in., because you cannot lean on a patient on a high couch, and it is therefore difficult to get any pressure behind your movements.

If you do not have a couch, a bed or mattress can be used for massage, but are not recommended. They are too wide to walk around, and far too bouncy: every time you put any pressure into a movement you merely compress the mattress springs and your patient is no better off! In the result you will tire yourself without accomplishing very much. A better idea is to find a table or desk which is long enough and not too high. Cover it with foam rubber or a few blankets and you will have a better working surface.

A good rule of thumb is to massage wherever you find a painful spot, all the while taking care not to hurt your patient unduly; if you are not sure about what you are doing, do not do it. The worst thing for a masseur to be is hesitant. If you decide to do something, do it, but if you convey a feeling of hesitation to your patient he will not feel safe in your hands, and his trust is something you need.

Your hands should be flexible, without being floppy. They should be extra-sensitive: use them to hear and see, as well as to feel. Keep your hands in contact with the skin in between movements if at all possible; this helps to keep up a constant flow. Do not talk to your patient unless he shows a desire to converse; even then let him lead the conversation. Talk to him with your hands.

It is difficult to dictate the speed at which massage should be done, but it is better to go slow rather than fast, so your hands can learn to feel as they pass over the skin. With practice they become sensitive to many things, but do not strain to feel. Massage slowly and rhythmically, with a clear, open mind. Certainly it is good to begin a massage with slow movements, but each massage you give is different, and the speed may vary as you go along.

It is very relaxing to massage in rhythm with your patient's breathing, or with your own breathing, or perhaps even both together. But do not force this if it does not happen naturally, otherwise it becomes contrived and does not feel right at all. With effleurage massage up the back as the patient breathes out, and come down again as he breathes in.

Every massage you give should be different, because every patient has different needs. Do not try to make each massage the same combination of movements in the same order, although working from a basic pattern.

Finally, do not give deep massage unless you have trained at a massage school: there are several good ones to choose from. Then you can be sure you are doing the right thing, in the correct way, for the right reason. Some basic ideas for body and facial massage oils are given in the recipes section.

Chapter 9

Skin Care

'For those secrets of nature, by which nature hath taught us how to beautifie, and make herself more comely, coming to my hands, I could not chuse but disperse them for the benefit of those to whom I owe so great a respect.'

Nicholas Culpeper

Perfuming the body with sweet scents and caring for the skin with natural oils is, perhaps, an indulgence, but it is a beautiful, innocent, and luxurious one. Like eating the 'fruits of trees and the grasses of the fields' it forms a part of our communion with nature; that is, as long as we use the products of nature. As perfumes essential oils are very simple, and have a naturalness that can never be imitated by synthetic perfumes. They are less sophisticated and less expensive, and many people find them an interesting alternative. Try rose and sandalwood, jasmine and bergamot, lavender and neroli, rose and geranium, or clary sage on its own. When giving treatment wiht an essence (or a blend of essences) it may be given to the patient to be worn as a perfume, if it appeals to them — a perfume and a remedy all in one!

Aromatics in general have a tradition of use in skin care which goes back some five thousand years, and perhaps even longer. The ancient Egyptians were probably the first to use aromatic toiletries to any extent. They made scented oils, unguents, and facial masks. They may have had some knowledge of distillation, but their scented oils were usually made by infusing aromatic herbs or gums in fatty oil. Unguents were made by similar infusions in heavy animal fat, or a mixture of oil and wax. Their masks contained such substances as powdered gums, pulverised herbs, honey, wax, oil, and so on. Their produced probably would not appeal to our more sophisticated tastes; we would find them a little too heavy, sticky, spicy, and resinous. But however they were scented these were the predecessors of modern skin care products and perfumes, and they were undoubtedly treasured by the Egyptian women who could afford them. Modern aromatherapy products, although in some ways more refined, are very similar to the old Egyptian recipes.

Just as orthodox medicine has become test-tube orientated, so modern cosmetics have become synthetic and unnatural. The swing back to more natural products can be seen as much in the toiletries trade as in foods and medicines. Products applied to the skin are often absorbed into the body, and affect it almost as much as those taken by mouth. For our own sakes, as well as for the sake of the thousands of animals killed annually in cosmetic laboratory experiments, we would do best to avoid highly synthetic products wherever possible. It is unfortunate that the word natural has been so over-used in advertising that it has ceased to mean anything, and is used to advertise even the most unnatural products.

Essential oils are an ideal form in which to use plants for skin care; they can easily be incorporated into any kind of base-creams, lotions, ointments, gels, toilet waters, perfumes, and so on. And of course most of them have an appealing scent. When giving a facial treatment the scent is important in itself, and when using essences it is possible to achieve a considerable degree of relaxation. Naturally enough the most pleasant scents are the most popular for skin care. In fact the flower oils seem to be the most useful — jasmine, rose, ylang-ylang, lavender, neroli, and camomile; their flowers are the most beautiful, and their oils the most beautifying.

> 'Applied to the skin these essences regulate the activity of the capillaries and restore vitality to the tissues. We might almost say that they make the flesh more succulent.'

The central theme of Mme Maury's book, *The Secret of Life and Youth*, is rejuvenation, and she suggests that essential oils are natural rejuvenating agents, and form a viable alternative to other methods. These 'other methods' usually involve some type of treatment with animal extracts — hormones, placentas, fresh cells, or the like. To me this type of therapy is barbaric; how can a product of death give new life? The subject of rejuvenation is a delicate one; man has always searched for the 'elixir of life'. Is it possible to regain lost youth, to add years to one's life? What is certainly possible is to improve one's general state of health, including that of the skin, so that one's appearance is improved, and along with it one's life expectancy. The only sure and safe way to do this is through natural health care and natural skin care, and in some cases the result is nothing short of rejuvenation. It depends on the state of the individual to begin with; if the person is relatively healthy, then the 'rejuvenation potential' is not very great. The pictures one sees in magazines of women who reduce from twenty stone to twelve stone are picture of rejuvenation.

Apart from the general process of improving one's health essential oils have a pronounced capacity to promote the elimination of waste matter and dead cells, and the regeneration of new, healthy cells. This applies whether they are used internally or applied to the skin, and is the main reason for their reputation as rejuvenating agents. They are well known for their antiseptic properties, and when regularly used will prevent decay and putrefaction. They were successfully used as embalming agents by many ancient civilisations, to preserve the flesh. Today they are used not only as antiseptics but also to prevent the growth of fungi, and as preservatives in both foodstuffs and cosmetics. It is easy to see why they are used to preserve youth. Maintaining a healthy body and a youthful complexion is at least as good, if not better, than rejuvenation, and the regular use of essential oils and aromatic skin care products is the surest and safest way to achieve this. For older people the more heavy essences, such as frankincense, sandalwood, and myrrh, are usually employed.

The ageing process cannot, of course, be slowed down or reversed, but rejuvenation in the sense of regaining lost health is the next best thing; indeed, would we really want our years back again? The ageing process of the skin is due to a number of factors. Wear and tear in a harsh environment, or chronic lack of health in the skin itself, encourage degeneration. Very dry or dehydrated skin will wrinkle more easily. The skin becomes flabby because it loses its elasticity and some of its subcutaneous fat. Chronic congestion of the skin (oiliness, pallor, blackheads, etc.), which is usually associated with general bodily congestion, leads to an excess of toxins (waste matter) in the cells of the lower layers of the skin. This causes an inefficient, unhealthy skin, and again the general ageing of the skin is speeded up. The antitoxic, antiseptic, and tonic properties of essences are of great value in preventing or clearing skin congestion.

Most, if not all, essences are cytophylactic; they stimulate the generation of new cells, and in so doing help to preserve the health and youth of the skin. This cytophylactic property is particularly evident in oils of lavender and orange blossom. It is one of the reasons why lavender oil is so good for healing burns, when the upper layers of the skin are destroyed. This was dramatically demonstrated to me when I was called on to treat a quite serious burn. The patient was a friend who lived nearby. He had taken the cap off his car radiator, not realising that the water was boiling. Immediately a powerful jet of steam shot up, searing his inner forearm, and taking off the whole of the epidermis, a severe second degree burn. He immediately rushed over to see me. I had never treated a serious burn in my life, and would have sent him to hospital, but I was working with a nurse who had plenty of casualty experience. She carefully removed the dead skin that was still stuck to his arm, and we treated it with fine gauze impregnated with neat lavender oil. The wound was extremely painful, but the essence stung only slightly, and then reduced the pain. At first he needed almost constant attention, but within seven days it was completely healed, with absolutely no scarring or hint of infection. My nurse was suitably impressed.

It is by no means necessary to use either lavender or neroli oil in every rejuvenating preparation. All essences share this property to some degree, and it is probably more useful to use essences on an individual basis, according to the personality and type of skin one is dealing with.

Hormone creams have a reputation for rejuvenating the skin. Fennel oil, which contains oestrogens, has a reputation as an anti-wrinkle agent. Other essences contain phytohormones, or have a hormonal action, which are of benefit in helping to rejuvenate the skin. Gattefossé comments that phytohormones have been found to benefit both dry and oily skins, and that they provoke a remarkable firming of the skin, stimulating the metabolism of the dermal cells, and acting as a rejuvenating active principle.

Essential oils are natural, organic substances, and work in harmony with the natural forces of the body. To make the most of aromatherapy, whether in skin care or health care, it is necessary to live according to the laws of nature, especially regarding food. The state of the skin so often reflects the state of the body, which in turn reflects the state of the mind. No amount of natural cosmetics and aromatics, however, will improve the skin as long as the diet consists of unnatural foods. Just as the skin needs protection from atmospheric pollution (dust, grit, coal smoke, etc.) it also needs protection from pollution from the inside. In this case the protection takes the form of careful eating. The health of the skin depends firstly on the blood, which nourishes it, and the health of the blood is largely determined by the food one eats. Secondly the health of the skin depends on the health and efficiency of the lymphatic system and extra-cellular fluid, as does every cell in the body. Overeating or wrong eating may lead to toxic congestion of these fluids, causing the skin (and other cells) to become slow and inefficient, and perhaps starving them of oxygen. Metabolic waste products gradually build up in the tissues causing congestion. Because the skin is an eliminative organ the body often tries to rid itself of these toxins through the skin, resulting in conditions such as acne. If the body is undernourished, which often happens in wrong eating, the skin will almost certainly be undernourished. A combination skin, which is oily in parts (usually on the forehead, nose and chin) and dry in other parts, may be the result of an overfed and undernourished body.

I have already indicated that it is difficult to treat the body by aromatherapy massage when the skin is in a very congested state, because absorption of the essences is greatly reduced. This is also a problem when treating the skin itself. One of the reasons why essential oils are so effective for treating skin problems is that they are readily absorbed by the skin, penetrating to the deepest levels of the dermis, and beyond. To avoid this congestion one should eat a reasonably non-toxic diet, free from chemical additives, low in sugar, salt, and 'foods' like chocolates, sweets, biscuits, cakes, coffee, alcohol, and so on. Grains, vegetables (raw or cooked), fruit, pulses, and vegetable protein may be freely eaten. If the body is undernourished a nutritional herbal tonic should be taken. This is more natural, and more easily absorbed by the body, than vitamin pills, and contains the necessary vitamins and minerals in a natural organic form.

When there is congestion a short fast, or fruit diet, followed by a change in diet will help considerably. It is not difficult to tell which people will respond best to a change in diet. Their foot reflexes to the stomach, intestines, and liver will be sore. Symptoms of toxic congestion are overweight, tiredness, sleeping too much, and skin eruptions. The people who most need a change in diet are those who live on cornflakes, hamburgers, cheese sandwiches, and coffee. The body needs time to adapt to a new internal environment, just as it does to a new external one; changes in diet should be gradual and long-lasting, rather than swift but short.

Certain skin conditions may be associated with deficiencies of one or more vitamins. I quote from *Let's Get Well* by Adelle Davis:

'Oily or dry skin. When volunteers have been kept on diets mildly lacking in vitamin B_2, the first symptoms were whiteheads and oily hair and skin. This condition cleared up soon after 5 to 15 milligrams of vitamin B_2 were given daily. To my knowledge, this abnormality has not been produced by any other deficiency.

'Dryness of the skin has resulted in volunteers lacking vitamins A, C, linoleic acid, or any one of several B vitamins. The oils of the skin are unsaturated and appear to be made almost wholly of the essential fatty acids; therefore unless vegetable oils are consumed, the skin is invariably dry.

'Stretch marks. Although healthy skin is amazingly elastic, previously overweight persons and most women who have had children retain stretch marks. This abnormality appears to result from the stress of inadequate reducing and pregnancy diets, which have allowed body proteins to be destroyed to the extent that scars have taken the place of weakened tissues.

'A friend who developed severe stretch marks during her first pregnancy stayed on an unusually high-protein diet supplement with 600 units of vitamin E and 300 milligrams of pantothenic acid daily through a subsequent pregnancy. Although she gave

birth to full-term twins, the stretch marks from the first pregnancy completely disappeared and none formed during the
second.'

As I have already hinted, the state of the body is affected by
the state of the mind. The skin is no exception; in fact the facial
skin is probably the clearest reflection of our states of mind, past
and present. Over the years grief, depression, anxiety, disgust,
fear, apathy, as well as joy, laughter, tenderness, and content-
ment, leave their mark. Our face is a mirror of our past life.
There is a world of difference between an aged, wrinkled face
that has happiness etched in it, and one which portrays nothing
but sadness and defeat. The difference may be between someone
who has had an easy life, and someone whose life has been
dogged with bad luck; or between the optimist and the pessimist,
not as regards what happens to us so much as how we react to it.
It is this state of mind, be it happy or sad, which shines through
so clearly in our face. Inner peace and happiness give even the
plainest features a life, a blossom, which no amount of make-up
or skin care can fake. A more obvious example is that of the
person with acne, who is so embarrassed by the condition that
she becomes tense and nervous inside, eats any food that is to
hand, and so perpetuates the condition.

The same destructive tendencies of grief, depression etc. constitute phychological factors in physical ill-health, and therefore
indirectly affect the state of one's skin. Excessive grief may affect
the heart, which may in turn cause redness or inflammation to
appear — not the heart bleeding, but the capillaries. This does
not mean that redness or broken veins are always the result of
grief, but it is obvious that the condition of the heart and blood
vessels affect the redness and blueness of the skin. Oils of neroli,
lavender, and sandalwood are primarily of use here, to bring a
soothing, calming, reassuring influence to skin, mind, and body.

Anger and frustration affect the liver: they inhibit its multiple
function. The result may be poorly assimilated food; you eat
enough, but your body does not incorporate as much of the
digested food as it should. This often leads to dry skin. Rose,
ylang-ylang, and rosemary will help to correct the imbalance of
the mind-body relationship, while rose, sandalwood, and
camomile will help the skin more directly. When dealing with
faulty digestion of any kind remember that most of the process of

149

digestion takes place in the small intestine, not the stomach, that digestive enzymes are produced by the gall bladder and pancreas (so the fault may lie with one of these), and that digestion begins in the mouth. The enzyme in the saliva converts cooked starch to sugar, so people with digestive problems must chew their food well, especially grains, potatoes, bread, etc. Poor assimilation is basically a problem of the liver, which plays a major part in the metabolism of proteins, fats, and carbohydrates. It also produces the bile secreted by the gall bladder, which aids the digestion of fats. Any form of alcohol, either internally or externally, should be avoided.

Anger and frustration will affect organs other than the liver, just as grief may affect not only the heart. There are as many different syndromes as there are shades of emotions. You know how your mouth dries up when you get a fright? Dehydrated skin is most often associated with fear, which correlates with the kidneys and bladder. It is the kidneys which regulate the amount of water in the body which, in turn, affects the water contents of the skin. A dehydrated skin may indicate a debydrated body, which may be due to insufficient fluid intake or to kidney malfunction. The main essences to use for this syndrome are clary sage, geranium, and sandalwood. There may be environmental factors to consider too, but as we all face much the same climatic and atmospheric conditions, the individual skin is usually the first consideration.

Oily skin is usually related physically to the large intestine, and emotionally to worry. Everybody worries to a certain degree, but real worriers tend to eat too much, choosing the wrong foods, especially chocolates, and drinking too much coffee. They probably also get constipated, because of the tension of thinking and worrying all the time. It is often very difficult to persuade these people to diet, but it is very important that they should. Oils of lavender, lemon, and geranium will help to check their condition, but a change in diet is nearly always essential to any real improvement. Mme Maure used to use a mixture of camomile, basil, and sandalwood as a systemic treatment for oily, congested skin.

The other type of skin, which is closely linked with oily skin, as dry is with dehydrated, is watery skin. This is also due to congestion, and results in puffiness. Obese people often have watery skins. This type correlates with the spleen, the lymphatic system, and the emotion of wonder, or compassion. They are slow, gullible, too kind, always wanting to help when their help is not needed. The use of lavender, rosemary, and juniper oil is indicated in this type.

To complete our examination of the effects of essential oils on the skin we should mention astringent oils, such as cypress and frankincense, which are an aid to healing when the skin is broken, such as in acne, and in discouraging the secretion of sebum in oily skin. As antiseptics they are of great value in cases of acne and infected seborrhoea (bergamot, juniper, lavender). The same oils may be used in seborrhoea of the scalp, which may manifest itself as oily hair or dandruff. The antiseptic effect is also related to their use as deodorants. They do not only cover up body odour, but inhibit the growth of the bacteria which cause it (bergamot, lavender, cypress).

We may also mention the opposing effects of stimulation and sedation, which also relate to the action of essences on the nervous system. The fact that an essence has a certain effect on the body internally does not necessarily mean that it has the same effect when applied to the skin, but in general this is the case.

Most essential oils stimulate or, if you prefer, irritate the skin, to varying degrees. Oils which are highly irritating, like mustard and wintergreen, may cause blistering or burning. Most oils are relatively mild irritants, and when sufficiently diluted their effect is beneficial, and no harm is done. However, if you use oils like camphor and eucalyptus neat on the skin you may cause irritation. If used on an already inflamed skin the result would be far from beneficial. For this reason it is unwise ever to use neat essences on the skin. When diluted, the stimulating effect of oils like juniper and camphor has the effect of increasing the local blood circulation. This is particularly useful for congested, toxic skin conditions which may result in acne, oily, or hydrated skin. However, stimulants should be tempered with emollients if there is inflammation, which is often the case with acne.

The emollient, cooling effect of oils such as camomile and rose is of value in all inflammatory conditions of the skin. Inflammation is usually due to infection or generally toxicity. These oils may also be used for sensitive skins and whenever there is redness or irritation. For redness due to highly sensitive or broken veins cypress oil should be combined with the sedative action of neroli. The effect of some oils on the blood, lymph, and the cells of the dermis also forms an important part of their general rejuvenating action. In this connection we may mention frankincense, myrrh, lavender, and neroli.

Generally speaking, essences should not be applied to the skin undiluted. To do so would be expensive, wasteful, and may not do the skin any good, except in those cases where a small amount of the essence is being used as a perfume.

The Skin

The skin, which has been called the largest organ in the body, covers an area of about 1.5 square metres. It covers every inch of you, keeping out cold, water, and undesirable organisms and substances, and keeping in heat, body fluids, and so on. It is the earth in which your hair and nails grow (and so the health of these three is intimately linked). It secretes sebum, a kind of waxy oil, which oils the hair. The sweat glands eliminate water-soluble waste products (sweat is very similar to urine; when you sweat a lot you do not urinate so much, and vice versa). On exposure to ultra-violet light substances called sterols in the skin are converted into vitamin D. (This is accompanied by an increase in pigmentation.) It also acts as a sense organ, recording touch, pressure, pain, heat, and cold.

The skin is also able to absorb certain substances, mainly those which are oil-soluble, such as essential oils.

Skin types
R. M. Gattefossé classified skin types into four major groups:

Oily
An excess of sebum, an oily, yellowish appearance, often large, dilated pores. Prone to acne and infection. The oil is most abundant where the sebaceous glands proliferate: the lower part of the nose, the chin, and the forehead.

Dry
Alipic — lacking in oil, but not necessarily dehydrated. A parchment-like appearance, often fragile in nature, with no apparent sebaceous gland openings, and related to a deficiency in endocrine secretion.

Dehydrated

Lacking in water — quickly wrinkled, drawn, often cold. Frequent in old people, and those exposed to the severities of the weather. Related to an endocrine imbalance — an excess of thyroid and a lack of adrenal secretion. People with this type of skin are often thin and emaciated.

Hydrated

Oedematic, having an excess of water; very sensitive to atmospheric variations. Sensitive to cold, and subject to chapping and chilblains. May be related to an abnormal viscosity of the blood, which slows up the circulation to the hands and feet.

This last type would appear to correspond to what we now call a 'sensitive' skin. It is interesting to note how these four skin types correspond with the four elements, and humours:

Sanguine	Phlegmatic	Choleric	Melancholic
Air	Water	Fire	Earth
Dry	Hydrated	Dehydrated	Oily

Gattefossé was also interested in astrology, and gives an astrological classification of skin types. He says that he finds this 'more readily usable than the scientific one, and it gives some interesting information on individual reactions'.

Mercury

A long face, fine chin, and spiritual eyes. The skin is generally fine and satin-like, but the face is mobile. The network of fine wrinkles, giving youth a joyous magnificence, soon shows up crow's feet and other wrinkles.

Venus

The skin is strong, but not tense, often covered with lanugo. The eyes are harder, yet more beautiful, and possibly less intelligent when the influence of Mercury is absent.

Earth

Has a squarish face, with angular lines, and an inelegant nose. Pronounced wrinkles, thick, tanned skin, which is scarcely softened by creams. Becomes like a shrivelled apple if the skin is dry, although it may also be oily.

Mars

Has a rectangular face, with horizontal, tufted eyes, thin lips, and a square chin. The skin is brown, and close. Wrinkles show up a relatively hard character. May develop facial hair with age.

Jupiter

A jovial type, hypothyroidal, with a tendency towards clamminess, and perhaps hirsuteness.

Saturn

Has a livid complexion, a sad appearance, with a sharp nose, drooping mouth, and arched eyebrows.

Sun

Has a cold, down-covered, sparkling, regularly fine, close-grained skin.

Moon

Has a round face, fresh-coloured, taut skin, finely grained, supple, and plump; arched lips, and a slender mouth.

These types do not necessarily correspond with one's birth sign, and mixed types are in the majority. Gattefossé comments that one should be able to distinguish the 'principal type' from the less dominant, 'parasitic type'. By eradicating the latter the woman's beauty is restored, as is the normal development of her underlying character. This is the way in which the old herbalists approached the humours. A certain humour is normally predominant in someone's personality; this is to be expected, and requires no treatment. It is when an abnormal balance of the humours comes about that treatment is required.

The ideal medium to use for both body and facial massage is a scented oil composed of vegetable oils and essences. Details of how to make these are given in the section on mixing and blending, and suggestions for facial massage are included in the massage section. The benefits of facial massage come from the massage itself as well as the essences used in the oil. Both are relaxing, but to obtain the maximum degree of relaxation the oils used should be appealing, and contain that extra quality that only the finest natural oils can give. You cannot expect someone to benefit fully from what is essentially a luxury treatment if they cannot smell luxury! If the blend is good and the patient likes the smell she will be able to relax and the success of your treatment is virtually assured.

The advantage of using vegetable oils for your massage is that they penetrate the skin much better than minerals oils, and yet do not penetrate so fast that you need repeatedly to apply more oil. The natural warmth produced by the massage opens the pores, thus aiding the penetration of the essences. A small amount of cream will be absorbed more quickly than an oil, although this also varies from one cream to another. Creams are ideal for quick individual applications but not for massage. After giving a facial massage the oil should be left on the skin for up to fifteen minutes, especially if the massage has been short. This gives the essences the time they need to penetrate and do their work. During this time warm compresses of plain or aromatic water should be laid over the whole area which has been massaged. The easiest way to do this is to use one piece of material such as white lint, with holes cut for the eyes and lower part of the nose. The eyes may then be covered with cucumber slices, or cotton wood pads impregnated with lavender or rose water. Eyes should always be kept slightly cooler than the rest of the face, and heat should not be applied to them for a period of time.

As an alternative to the compress you may use a facial steamer or atomiser. This is especially good for acneic or congested skins, as it is more stimulating and extractive than a compress; you may use an atomiser for any type of skin, with two or three drops of an appropriate essence or blend of essences added to the water. After using your compress or atomiser (you could, of course, use one and then the other) you will be surprised how well the oils have penetrated, and it should not be necessary to cleanse the skin at this point. If there is still a trace of oil just dab lightly with a tissue. The really deep cleansing process takes place with your next application — the face pack, or facial mask.

There are several basic ingredients which you will need for any mask. These include yoghurt, kaolin or fuller's earth, fruit or vegetable oil, and essential oils. Yoghurt is cleansing, toning, extractive, and mild enough to be used on any skin. Always use plain, live yoghurt, because its action largely depends on the bacteria it contains. Yoghurt, like fruit pulp, is too slippery to use on its own; it just slides off the face, so you need to mix it with powdered clay (kaolin or fuller's earth) or some other powder

155

such as fine oatmeal. The yoghurt-clay mixture can be used as a base for any mask.

The more dry, dehydrated type of skin requires a mild, moisturising, nutritional mask, for which fruit is ideal. The fruit should be peeled and then pulped either by hand or in a blender. You may alternatively use just the fruit juice, but pulp is preferable; as a moisturiser add honey. The fruit pulp is added to the basic mixture, together with a little wheat-germ oil, in the case of dry or mature skin, and two to three drops of essential oil. In the case of congested, acneic, oily types of skin the clay powder should predominate. These clays have strong anti-toxic properties and are excellent extractive agents, drawing impurities out from the skin. Brewer's yeast may be added to enhance the extractive process, along with grape or cabbage juice. To summarise:

Acne	Cabbage, grape, tomato, yeast, camphor, juniper, bergamot
Oily	Cabbage, grape, lemon, pear, strawberry, camphor, frankincense
Sensitive	Honey and yoghurt, grape, melon, neroli, rose, camomile
Dry	Avocado, banana, carrot, melon, wheat-germ oil, rose, sandalwood
Mature	Apple, avocado, grape, lemon, wheat-germ oil, cypress, frankincense, patchouli
Hydrated	Clay, oatmeal or linseed meal, juniper, lavender
Normal	Avocado, grape, lemon, peach, wheat-germ oil, jasmine, neroli, lavender

Let me emphasise that this is a summary and it is not necessary to use all the ingredients mentioned under each heading. You only need one or two fruits and one or two essences in each case. For a normal skin your could use any fruits and almost any oils. If you find it impractical to pulp the fruits, you can simple use clay powder, yoghurt, and essences. The essential oils I have mentioned here are well-tried suggestions, but other oils may be used in each case.[1] The face mask is

1 See Therapeutic Index, p. 307.

primarily nourishing and extractive. It stimulates local blood circulation, promotes the elimination of waste material, and continues the work which was started by the facial massage. At the same time it may be soothing and moisturising, according to the ingredients used. By using fresh fruits and yoghurt, which are both live and organic, and by using them in conjunction with the dynamic action of essences one is often able to produce results which can only be described as rejuvenating. But remember, once is not enough, and lasting results will only be obtained by regular use of masks. A normal skin only needs a mask every one or two weeks.

The mask should be left for up to twenty minutes to complete its task, after which time it should be gently sponged off with tepid water. You may at this point apply a compress or, preferably, an atomiser with essences to tone and refresh the skin, and to encourage the pores to close; cypress, juniper, or bergamot oils may be used. The skin should now be tissue-dried and, if desired, a little moisturising cream may be very gently patted into the skin. If you have a moisturising cream base you can add your own essences to it, making your own creams for each different skin type. Use pots which have a good seal, otherwise the oils, which are not incorporated during the manufacturing process will tend to evaporate. You can also make your own cleansing creams, soothing creams, and so on in this way. Alternatively a commercial product may be used. No make-up of any kind should be used after a facial treatment of this type, because it will largely undo the benefit of the treatment; the skin must be allowed to breathe.

Chapter 10

Practical Hints and Recipes

Quantities and Dilutions

These are all given in ml (millilitres). For the purposes of this book 1 ml, 1 cc (cubic centimetre) and 1 g (gramme) may be regarded as interchangeable.

$$1 \text{ ml} = 20 \text{ Drops}$$
$$5 \text{ ml} = 1 \text{ tsp.}$$
$$30 \text{ ml} = 1 \text{ fl. oz.}$$
$$500 \text{ ml} = 1 \text{ pint}$$
$$1,000 \text{ ml} = 1 \text{ litre}$$

Massage Oils

For all massage oils, whether face or body, we use a dilution of 2½%. This happens to be a very convenient dilution, because it is equivalent to: ONE DROP OF ESSENCE TO EVERY 2 ml OF VEGETABLE OIL.

For example, a typical blend would look like this:

	%	ml
Essential oil	2½	1.25 = 25 drops
Almond oil	97½	48.75
	100%	50 ml

Notice that there are *25* drops of essence to *50 ml* of total blend. Whatever size of bottle you are using, simply divide its capacity in mls by 2, and this will give you the total number of drops of essential oil for that bottle. Do not worry about measuring vegetable oil exactly. First add drops of essential oil to the bottle, and then just fill up to the top with your vegetable oil.

Ointments

For ointments we use twice the concentration of essential oil —
5%. This means that the total amount in mls is *the same* as the
number of drops of essence. For example:

	%	ml	
Essential oil	5	1.5	= 30 drops
Almond oil	75	22.5	
Beeswax	20	6 g	
	100%	30 ml	

See following text for how to go about making your ointments.

Inhalations

  8 – 12 drops for bowl of hot water
  4 – 6 drops for facial steamer
  See following text.

Baths

  3 – 5 drops of essential oil
  See p. 108.

Compresses

  2 drops of essential oil to 1 pint of warm water.
  See p. 114.

When prescribing oils for therapeutic use the total pattern of the
patient's symptoms should be considered. Consult the
Therapeutic Index for each symptom or condition, and note the
oils which most often apply. Then consult the section on
Essences which deals with each of your short list of oils. You
will find one or more essences which seem to be appropriate.
Very often one essence is sufficient, in which case use that.
Treatment is not necessarily improved by using a blend of
several essences, and if one oil fits the case perfectly no useful
purpose is served by combining it with other oils.

   If there is no one essence which seems to cover most of the
symptoms it will be necessary to blend several together, but try to
keep them to a minimum, say between two and five oils. The
resulting blend is not simply a combination of the properties of
its ingredients; it has its own individual properties, as if you had
created a new essential oil. Although there are only twenty-eight
essences described in this book the permutations of combinations
of either three, four, or five essences come to over twelve million.

159

In traditional Chinese herbal medicine certain basic rules were followed which are included here for interest; I have found some of them very useful. Illnesses caused by the action of cold on the body should be subdued with hot medicines; cold medications should be administered for illnesses caused by heat. Medicines for ailments above the chest should be taken after meals. Medicines for ailments below the heart and stomach should be taken before meals. Medicines for sickness in the four limbs should be taken early in the morning on an empty stomach; for afflictions of bones and marrow, in the evening after a meal.

Medicinal herbs were divided into four categories: 'emperor' herbs (the principal curative agent), 'minister' herbs (a synergist, or adjuvant, aiding the action of the 'emperor'), 'chancellor' herbs (which set the healing process in motion, having a catalytic effect), and 'ambassadors' which were vehicles or bases for the prescription. Prescriptions themselves were based on the 'doctrine of the seven recipes', in which recipes were categorised as follows:

1. *Ch'i fang*, or odd-numbered recipe, containing an odd number of ingredients. This is basically a yang recipe, and is prescribed only for yin conditions.
2. *Go fang*, or even-numbered recipe. A yin recipe, containing an even number of ingredients.
3. *Ta fang*, or great recipe. A very powerful recipe, used only for serious illnesses, and usually when there are many symptoms.
4. *Hsao fang*, or little recipe. Used in simple illnesses, where there are only one or two symptoms. Only two or three ingredients are used.
5. *Huan fang*, or slow recipe. A relatively mild recipe, used for patients in a very weak state, whose condition could not stand up to strong drugs. This recipe builds strength.
6. *Chi fang*, or emergency recipe. A prescription with an immediate effect, often used for patients near to death.
7. *Ch'ung fang*, or repeated recipe. Used for complicated illnesses which affect several different organs. Contains many ingredients, and is taken over a period of time.

In homoeopathic medicine it is not really necessary to make a classical medical diagnosis, and homoeopaths are sometimes scornful of such diagnosis. The drug picture, the pattern of symptoms, is of prime importance. It is not necessary to know whether the patient has asthma or bronchitis, but it is very important to prescribe the correct remedy. In acupuncture it is also essential to make a correct diagnosis, although it is not done along Western medical lines.

In aromatherapy the general state of the patient should be taken into account, and even apparently insignificant symptoms may help in prescribing the correct remedy. However, this is not done to the same extent as in homoeopathy, and a correct ortho- dox diagnosis is also important. It is very easy to consult the Therapeutic Index once you know what the problem is, but you must be sure of what you are treating.

Once a diagnosis has been made and the appropriate remedy or remedies selected, they may be applied either externally or inter- nally, or both. Taking oils orally is not necessarily more effective than applying them externally. For internal use they should be taken in honey water. For one dose dissolve 1 teaspoon of honey in 30 ml (1 fl. oz.) of very warm water. Add the drops of essential oil and swallow. Always take your oils after eating.

Ill-health, it should be remembered, is never purely physical; it always involves some psychological element. As far as possible, therefore, we want the oils we blend for massage to smell appeal- ing. If, by merely altering the relative percentage of each oil in the mixture, we can improve its scent appeal, we are gaining much and losing nothing. One instinctively shies away from using large quantities of strong oils, and of course is right in doing so. When it comes to blending, our nose is our best guide. People often ask if there are any oils which should never be mixed; there are not. But the best way to judge whether two particular oils harmonise is to mix them and smell. You will find that certain oils har- monise better than others; also that there is a ratio, a proportion, in which they blend better than any other. It may take a little time to find the balance but you will learn best from experience. After you have tried a number of blends you will know what propor- tions to use in almost any given mixture.

Massage Oils

When mixing an oil for external use there are two basic ingre- dients: essential oil and vegetable oil (known, in this context, as a 'carrier oil'). The carrier oil acts as a vehicle for the blend of essences, so they can be diluted to a desirable strength, and can

161

be applied as an ordinary massage oil. Your choice of vegetable oil will be ruled partly by price, but there are other considerations. If you want an oil which will nourish the skin, as well as acting as a vehicle, avocado pear and wheat-germ oils are particularly rich in vitamins. They are, however, rather heavy to use on their own, and can be mixed with a lighter vegetable oil, so that your 'carrier' is nourishing but not too heavy. I find sweet almond oil best for general use, but olive, soya bean, or sunflower seed can all be used.

Another important consideration is that nearly all vegetable and essential oils oxidise: they go rancid. The result is an unpleasant odour in vegetable oils, and a distinct loss of freshness and worsening of odour in essential oils. The oils end up by going cloudy, and their therapeutic value is considerably reduced. Once oxidation has set in it is a process which cannot be reversed. This is why it is important to keep oils in air-tight containers, preferably well filled, and never to put fresh oil into a used bottle. Fortunately nature has provided us with a natural anti-oxidant in the form of wheat-germ oil: this is due to its high vitamin E content. Always include 5% to 10% of wheat-germ oil in your blends. They will not last for ever, but will keep longer than usual; exactly how long depends on how often the bottle is opened, but five months is the average period, if the oils are fresh to begin with.

The quantity of essential oil to use depends a little on the strength of the essences, but I suggest 2% for general use. Essences are very powerful, and you only need to use just enough. Do not think that if you use more oil you will get better or quicker results. The percentage of essence in the plant varies between 0.01% and about 10%. The average is between 1% and 2%.

I have heard many strange tales about blending oils, as if it was some kind of witchcraft, but it is really very simple. It is not necessary to warm them, unless they are solid at room temperature. It is not necessary to do it on a full moon at midnight where seven ley-lines meet! You simple fill your bottle with vegetable oil (or oils), then add the essences by drops. Cap the bottle and shake gently. I know some people prefer to mix each essence with an appropriate amount of vegetable oil (say, 2% mixtures) and then use these mixtures for blending. This is certainly possible, although your oils are likely to go rancid much more quickly than if you keep the essences separate until blending.

If you want your oils to keep their scent for the maximum possible time, both in the bottle and out, they will need to be well 'fixed'. In other words your blend must include at least one oil from the lower third of the volatility rate table. Fixatives are used in perfumery to help delay the evaporation of the perfume, so that the scent lasts longer, and also so that the fragrance does not change too much as it evaporates. Sandalwood oil is the best all-round fixative for scent, although patchouli, myrrh and cedar-wood are also very effective.

Although essential oils are expensive to buy, it is impractical to think of distilling one's own. You need several hundredweight of herbs, and specialised equipment, and a considerable amount of technical knowledge. However, there is another process, much easier to do, which herbalists were doing hundreds of years ago:

> 'Oyle of roses is made thus. Some boyle roses in oyle and kepe it, some do fyll a glasse with roses and oyle and they boyle it in a caudron full of water and this oyle is good. Some stampe fresh roses with oyle and they put it in a vessel of glasse and set it in the sune IIII dais and this oyle is good.'

> 'Oyle of voylettes is made thus. Sethe vyolettes in oyle and streyne it. It will be oyle of vyolettes.'

These oils, which the French perfumers used to call *huiles antiques* and which I call 'infused oils', are not much used for perfumes, internal medicines, inhalations, or aromatic waters, but they are very good for aromatherapy massage. The result is similar to mixing vegetable and essential oils. There are basically two methods. One is to put herb and oil in a well-sealed container, which is then placed in a saucepan with two or three inches of water in the bottom. The water is then boiled for an hour, and the oil heated without actually boiling. Oil and herb are then separated by straining, and a fresh portion of herbs mixed with the oil, which is then heated again. You can do this as many times as you like, and each time the oil will get stronger. The stronger the oil, the more you will need to dilute it for use in massage. The other method is to place herbs and oil in a clear glass container, and leave it in strong sunlight, changing the herbs every two to three days. Although essences should not be exposed to light, this method seems to produce oils of very good quality. I feel sure that the sunlight must charge the oil with so much energy that any negative aspects as nullified. Most herbs need a little bruising first so that the essence mixes easily with the fatty oil.

CHAPTER 10
Ointments, Waters, Inhalations

Ointments are very easy to make. All you need is essence, oil, and wax, blended in the correct proportions. I always use beeswax (the yellow is more natural than the white). The wax has to be melted before it will mix with the oil, and you will need about one part beeswax to four parts of oil. Heat oil and wax together in a dish placed in pan of hot water. When the wax melts, take away the dish from the heat. As the mixture first begins to solidify round the sides add the essences, stir, and pour it into containers. Then put the containers in a cold-water bath to speed up the cooling process. The reason for adding the essence at the last minute is to ensure that as little as possible evaporates before the ointments solidifies. For a softer ointment use five parts oil, one part beeswax, and one part vaseline. If you include wheat-germ oil, and keep in well-sealed pots, your ointments will last up to a year. A scented ointment, by the way, is known as a pomade. All the earliest perfumes, balms, and cosmetic unguents were made in the form of pomades.

A very simple way of making fragrant waters is to mix a few drops of essence with distilled water. By this method you can make waters of rose, orange blossom, lavender, geranium, indeed of any essence you like. By mixing several essences you can make up some fine blended toilet waters, following the recipes given at the end of this chapter. Use about one drop of essence per half cup of distilled water. As this mixture must be kept air-tight it is best to use a bottle, for example a baby's bottle with an air-tight cap. Add two or three drops of essence to 100 ml. of distilled water, replace the cap and shake vigorously. Although the essence does not dissolve completely it is dispersed sufficiently to produce a satisfactory aromatic water. If stored properly these waters will keep for several weeks. If sufficient alcohol is added a true solution will be obtained, but alcohol is not very good for the skin; indeed alcohol suitable for this purpose is impossible to obtain.

Essences, blended oils, or other preparations should always be kept in cool, dry, dark, air-tight conditions.

For inhalations between eight and twelve drops of essence should be used. Sprinkle on to the surface of a bowl of hot water (between one and two pints). The water should be boiled, poured out, and then left to cool for one minute before adding the essences. If it is too hot the vapours of the oils are a little too strong to inhale. An alternative method is to use a facial steamer, again placing the essences in the water. This is a neater method because the water is kept at a constant temperature, and half the amount of essential oil is required. Inhale slowly and deeply for five to ten minutes; the traditional towel over the head is not strictly necessary.

Details of baths and compresses are given in the chapter on baths.

Cosmetic and Medicinal Oils

Facial Oils

For normal skin

Geranium	6 drops
Jasmine	3 drops
Lavender	16 drops
	25

For dry skin

Geranium	7 drops
Rose	4 drops
Sandalwood	14 drops
	25

For oily skin

Bergamot	12 drops
Cypress	8 drops
Juniper	5 drops
	25

For inflamed or sensitive skin

Rosewood	12 drops
Neroli	4 drops
Rose	4 drops
	20

NOTE: In each case the 25 drops should be diluted in 50 ml of vegetable oil.

Skin Tonic Waters

Normal skin	Bergamot	4 drops
	Jasmine	10 drops
Dry skin	Geranium	10 drops
	Rose	7 drops
Acne	Bergamot	10 drops
	Lavender	6 drops
Oily skin	Cypress	7 drops
	Juniper	10 drops

Use distilled water if possible. The above figures, in drops, will make 50 ml of aromatic water.

Hair Care

For loss of hair

Juniper	7 drops
Lavender	9 drops
Rosemary	9 drops
	25 drops

For greasy hair or dandruff

Cedarwood	7 drops
Cypress	9 drops
Juniper	9 drops
	25 drops

These should be made up in a 2½% dilution in vegetable oil. Massage well into the scalp and leave on for at least one hour. Apply shampoo to hair and rub in before adding water, otherwise oil is difficult to remove.

Hand Care

For dry or chapped hands

Make up an ointment or oil using the following recipe:

Benzoin
Patchouli   } equal parts
Rose

Massage well into hands for at least two minutes. It is best to do this at night, and then go to bed wearing an old pair of cotton gloves.

Perspiring hands

Use hand baths, as for perspiring feet. You may also use as a compress, or simply pat in a little aromatic water.

Baths

Quantities for one bath

For a hangover

Fennel	1 drop
Juniper	2 drops
Rosemary	1 drop
	4 drops

May also be applied in compresses to liver and head. This bath is also useful for obesity.

For nervous exhaustion

Basil	1 drop
Geranium	2 drops
Lavender	2 drops
	5 drops

167

Foot Baths

For perspiring feet

Clary	2 drops
Cypress	3 drops
Lavender	2 drops
	7 drops

For tired, aching feet

Juniper	3 drops
Lavender	2 drops
Rosemary	2 drops
	7 drops

Hip Baths

For haemorrhoids

Cypress	3 drops
Frankincense	2 drops
Juniper	2 drops
	7 drops

For impotence, frigidity

Clary sage	6 drops
Jasmine	1 drop
	7 drops

Douches

For leucorrhoea

Bergamot	1 drop
Lavender	3 drops
Rose	1 drop
	5 drops

(Hyssop, juniper, or sandalwood may also be taken internally.)

For painful periods

Clary	2 drops
Marjoram	2 drops
Camomile	1 drop
	5 drops

Irregular or scanty menstruation

Clary	2 drops
Melissa	2 drops
Rose	1 drop
	5 drops

Vaginal pruritis

Bergamot	2 drops
Camomile	1 drop
Peppermint	1 drop
	4 drops

Each recipe should be diluted in a pint of water.

Massage Oils

For rheumatic pain

Frankincense	5 drops
Eucalpytus	5 drops
Rosemary	15 drops
	25 drops

To tone muscles and relieve mild aches

Juniper	6 drops
Lavender	12 drops
Rosemary	7 drops
	25 drops

A generally relaxing oil

Geranium	10 drops
Lavender	10 drops
Marjoram	5 drops
	25 drops

An aphrodisiac oil

Rosewood	13 drops
Jasmine	4 drops
Ylang-ylang	8 drops
	25 drops

NOTE: In each case the 25 drops should be diluted in 50 ml of vegetable oil.

Antiseptics

An antiseptic mouth wash

Bergamot	2 drops
Lavender	1 drop

Dilute in a cup of water.

An antiseptic ointment for cuts, etc.

Essences

Bergamot	12 drops
Eucalyptus	4 drops
Lavender	14 drops
	30 drops

Base

Vaseline	1 oz	30g

or

Vegetable oil	1 oz	30 g
Beeswax	¼ oz	7 g

Heat ointment base until it melts, add essences, stir, pour into jar, and cool rapidly.

The same essences may be used, diluted in water, as an antiseptic wash for cuts, sores, etc.

Disinfecting air freshener

Bergamot	155 drops
Eucalyptus	5 drops
Juniper	40 drops
	200 = 10 ml

Mix essences, and keep in a dropper bottle. Use as a general air freshener, also in sick rooms, toilets, etc. May also be used as a disinfectant for washing floors and furniture, nappies, putting down drains, and so on.

Inhalations

For head cold or other condition with blocked sinuses

Basil	2 drops
Eucalyptus	7 drops
Peppermint	1 drop
	10 drops

For influenza or heavy colds with fever

Camphor	3 drops
Eucalyptus	7 drops
	10 drops

For bronchitis, etc. as an expectorant/antiseptic

Bergamot	3 drops
Eucalyptis	3 drops
Sandalwood	4 drops
	10 drops

For asthma, bronchitis as an antispasmodic

Hyssop	2 drops
Lavender	6 drops
Marjoram	2 drops
	10 drops

Medicinal Oils

For spasmodic cough

Cypress	2 drops
Hyssop	3 drops

For indigestion or colic

Basil	1 drop	Juniper	2 drops
Cardamom	1 drop	Peppermint	1 drop

For gall stones

Bergamot	2 drops		
Eucalyptus	1 drop	*or* Rosemary	2 drops

For urinary stones

Camomile	2 drops
Geranium	2 drops
Juniper	2 drops

Each recipe should be taken three times daily in honey water — see p. 319.

Some Recipes from 'Arts Master-Piece or the beautifying part of Physick' by Nicholas Culpeper

A sweet water of the Italians, which they call damask-water

Take of cynamon one ounce, cloves half an ounce, sweet-marjoram, rosemary, lavender, bay-leaves, pennyroyal, green province roses, each a handful, mallego wine, rose water, each a pint and a half, cut the green things, powder the dry ones, and set them in the sun six dayes, then distill them in a double vessel; some add to them citron pill, storax calamite, orrice, each one dram, and flowers of jasmine, they sprinkle this water on their garments, linnen, hands, and nostrils.

A sweet-scented bath for noble-women

Take of roses, citron pill, citron flowers, orange flowers, jasmine, bays, rosemary, lavender, mint pennyroyal, spring water, each a sufficient quantity, boyl them together gently, and make a bath, to which adde oyl of spike five drops, musk five grains, ambergreece three grains, sweet asa one ounce, let her go into the bath two hours before meat.

Another to cleanse the body and make it comely

Take of sage, lavender-flowers, rose-flowers, each two handfulls, a little salt, boyl them in water, or in a lye, and make a bath not too hot, in which bathe the body two hours before meat.

A water against blood-shed eyes

Take of benjamin one ounce, pure white honey half a pint, fennel and rue water each twelve drams, water of sweet marjoram half an ounce, distill them in an alembick.

A sweet ointment

Take oyl of nutmeg made by a press, one dram, the best sivet one scruple, choice musk six granes, oyl of spike, oyl of lavender, each two drops or three, make an ointment, to anoint the forehead, nostrils, and other principal parts, to fortifie them.

An ointment to whiten the hands
Take of pine-nuts cleansed and bruised, one pound, mustard-seed one ounce, figs three ounces, camphure two drams, beat them all well and mix them, and make a paste to rub the hands.

To keep the breasts small
Take of roche-alume poudered a sufficient quantity, oyl of roses as much as is sufficient, mix them and anoint the breasts.

An oyl to cure a red face
Take four ounces of peach kernels, goard-seed two ounces, bruise them and make an oyl to anoint the face morning and evening.

Oyls to take away the wrinkles of the face
Oyl of turkey-millett, and the decoction of its berries, do distend, mollifie, and consolidate wrinkles; also oyl of nuts is good.

Oyl of southernwood doth produce hair
It is made as oyl of rue, it is good to cause hair to grow; and in shedding of hair it is anointed with labdanum and bears fat.

An ointment for the clefts of the nibbles (cracked nipples)
Take oyl of roses, the middle rind of elder, each one ounce, wax as much as is sufficient, mix them.

Some Miscellaneous Recipes

These two recipes are from entirely different sources:

Aqua aromatica

Cinnamon bark	3 parts	Sage leaves	10 parts
Lavender flowers	5 parts	Fennel seeds	3 parts
Peppermint leaves	5 parts	Spirit	70 parts
Rosemary leaves	5 parts	Water	300 parts

Aqua mirabilis

Cinnamon oil	1 part	Sage oil	1 part
Lavender oil	1 part	Fennel oil	1 part
Peppermint oil	1 part	Spirit	350 parts
Rosemary oil	1 part	Water	644 parts

A book of recipes, published in 1681, states that *aqua mirabilis* 'suffereth not the heat to burne not melancholy nor flegme to be lift up or to have dominion above nature, it also expells reumes and profiteth a good colour, keepth and preserveth visage and ye memory . . .'

Bruise oil

Camomile, feverfew, betony, lavender, melissa, rosemary, sage, rosebuds, southernwood, wormwood.

Take of each a handful and chop them small, put in a stone jar with sufficient salad oil to cover them. Stand for a fortnight, stirring often. Then boil gently till the oil is extracted, but do not exceed the heat of boiling water. Strain through linen, and keep in a well-corked bottle.

Emollient skin balm

Quince seed	½ oz	Oil of bay	10 drops
Water	7 oz	Oil of cloves	5 drops
Glycerine	1½ oz	Oil of orange peel	10 drops
Alcohol	4½ oz	Oil of wintergreen	8 drops
Salicylic acid	6 grains	Oil of roses	2 drops
Carbolic acid	10 grains		

Digest the quince seed in the water for twenty-four hours, and then press through a cloth. Dissolve the salicylic acid in the alcohol; add the carbolic acid to the glycerine; put all together, shake well, and bottle.

175

Mouth wash

Quillaia bark	125 parts	Glycerine	95 parts
Alcohol	155 parts		

Macerate for four days, then add:

Acid. carbol.		Ol. roseae	0.6 part
cryst	4 parts	Ol. cinnam.	0.6 part
Ol. geranii	0.6 part	Tinct. ratanhae	45 parts
Ol. caryophyll	0.6 part	Aqua rosae	900 parts

Macerate again for four days and filter.

Eau-de-Cologne

Rosemary oil	5 parts	Lavender oil	5 parts
Neroli oil	20 parts	Bergamot oil	220 parts
Lemon oil	75 parts	Alcohol 90%	5,000 parts

Carmelite balm water

Melissa oil	30 minims	Clove	15 minims
Marjoram oil	3 minims	Coriander oil	5 minims
Cinnamon oil	10 minims	Angelica oil	3 minims
Lemon oil	30 minims	Alcohol 90%	10 fl oz

Florida water

Bergamot oil	3 fl oz	Neroli oil	½ fl oz
Clove oil	1¼ fl dr	Jasmine oil	6 fl oz
Cinnamon oil	2½ fl oz	Rose water	1 pint
Lavender oil	1 fl oz	Alcohol	8 pints
Lemon oil	1 fl oz		

Chapter 11

The Essential Oils

This chapter includes the following essential oils:

Basil	Hyssop
Benzoin	Jasmine
Bergamot	Juniper
Black pepper	Lavender
Camomile	Marjoram
Camphor	Melissa
Cardamom	Myrrh
Cedarwood	Orange blossom (Neroli)
Clary sage	Patchouli
Cypress	Peppermint
Eucalpytus	Rose
Fennel	Rosemary
Frankincense	Sandalwood
Geranium	Ylang-ylang

Classifying essences as yin or yang inevitably projects a limited concept onto something which is very dynamic in its action. Every essence has both yin and yang qualities, and its predominating effect also depends on the circumstances of its application. However, reference to the yin-yang quality of an oil provides a key from which an understanding of that oil's therapeutic action can be built up; it also provides a useful tool for comparing essences.

The same applies to the use of astrological classification. Although I do not enlarge on the use of astrology in prescribing oils, the information is here included for those who wish, and are able, to use it. Although in most cases I have used Culpeper as a reference for the ruling planets, some of the plants in this book were not known to him. The planets ascribed to these were selected on the basis of my own knowledge of the four elements.

The indexes of evaporation rate and odour intensity are taken from the work of Louis Appell. The odour intensity rates are in a scale of 1 to 10, but none of the oils falls below the figure 4. This is because the original study included aromatic chemicals, some of which are rated lower than 4. Relatively speaking, then, essences with an intensity of 7 have a medium intensity, and those rated at 4 have the lowest intensity. The evaporation rates are in a scale of 1 to 100. Thus eucalyptus oil has the highest evaporation rate (5) and patchouli the lowest (100). These figures are different from the ones actually used by Louis Appell, but the relative values are the same. Most of these evaporation rates are different from those obtained by W. A. Poucher before the war. Poucher used a much more subjective method, and inevitably took odour intensity into account at the same time. I have also included a table of his figures, because they may be useful for distinguishing top, middle, and base notes. Some of the essences in this book were not included in Appell's work. In these cases I have either given a figure, followed by a query, or left a blank.

Those who are familiar with the ways of science know how difficult it is to prove anything of a general nature. This is especially true of living organisms. Experiments with drugs are performed on cats, rats, mice, dogs, guinea pigs and, occasionally, human beings. Quite often the results of two different experiments will be contradictory; one may demonstrate that a certain drug raises the blood pressure, and another that it lowers blood pressure. This is why such experiments have become more and more rigid in the control of every condition. In the above example, for instance, did they use exactly the same substance, in the same dose, for the same length of time, on the same species of animal, applied in the same way? Other factors, such as the time of year, time of day, geographical location, the astrological influence of the stars, the state of mind of the animal, and the attitude of the scientist towards the experiment, may well influence its outcome. Some of these factors have been shown by Lyall Watson in *Supernature* to have such an influence.

As the controls of an experiment become more and more rigid, it becomes increasingly difficult to interpret and apply its results. We can say that, given the exact conditions — location, animal used, dose, etc. — a certain result was obtained. But how significant is that result, and how useful? Because it was true in those conditions, will it be true in others? Because cinnamon oil was demonstrated to stimulate the heart muscle of a dog, which was anaesthetised, and had its chest cut open, in the USA in 1962, does that mean that, for us, cinnamon oil is a heart stimulant?

The scientist assumes that if two experiments obtain contradictory results there must be a logical reason: at least one of the conditions must have been different. He assumes that, logically, a substance should always have the same effect, given the same conditions. This may well be true, but we must be sure to include all conditions, including astrological ones, and the fact is that the latter never repeat themselves exactly.

When the scientist has done away with enough dogs and cats, and is satisfied that his drug had certain properties, and is not too toxic, he turns his attention to human beings, in what are called clinical trials. When the drug has been properly tested out on us, it may be given the seal of approval, and put on the market. Every so often a drug like hexachloraphene or thalidomide is found, some years later, to be dangerous, and is taken off the market. So even when a substance has been in clinical use for a number of years, we cannot be certain that it is safe to use. And 'safe' is only a relative consideration; is any drug totally safe to use?

There are a small number of essential oils, such as wormwood, which are classed as toxic, and a very large amount (10 – 20 ml) taken by mouth would probably have fatal consequences. However, these toxic oils are not on general sale. The oils which are available are non-toxic, and even an overdose would be relatively harmless. At least with essences you can be sure that you are not suddenly going to develop a brand new disease. Most essences have been in use now for over a hundred years, and many of them for four hundred years or longer. The ones that have been dropped from pharmacopoeias were dropped because of their relative mildness, not because they were found to be dangerous. Many essences actually show anti-toxic properties, counteracting poisoning from substances such as snake venom, barbiturates, or alcohol.

Many impressive tests and experiments have been done with oils, and a number of informative articles have been published.

Much of what is said supports the empirical uses to which the same aromatics were put by the old herbalists. This, for me, is more convincing than isolated experiments on animals. The test of time is not so much a test of therapeutic power, but of therapeutic integrity. Most of the results confirm the empirical uses of the oil. Where they do not, or where there is disagreement or other reasons for uncertainty, one can only rely on intuition, developing an understanding of the oil, by consulting the old herbals, examining the plant in its wild state (if possible), and noting its colours, structure, and 'vibration'. By getting to know every quality of an oil and its parent plant, one can feel whether or not a certain property forms part of its character.

I have found it difficult when writing about each oil, to distinguish between properties or uses gleaned from old herbals, and those based on modern experiments. Often they overlap, and when they do not, who can say which is right? In painting the picture I have sometimes applied a few brush strokes from my own experience or intuition, although I have tried to be as factual as possible. I have quoted extensively from older herbals, not only for their interest value but as a part of the information given for each oil. Sometimes the original text can convey so much more than a paraphrase, or contains minor details not included in my own summary or the Therapeutic Index.

Basil

Latin name	Ocimum basilicum
Family	Labiatae
Quality	Yang
Ruling planet	Mars
Evaporation rate	78
Odour intensity	7
Essence from	Herb

Properties

Antidepressant
Antiseptic
Antispasmodic
Carminative
Cephalic
Digestive
Emmenagogue
Expectorant
Febrifuge
Nervine
Stimulant of
   adrenal cortex
Stomachic
Sudorific
Tonic

Uses

Bronchitis
Cold (chronic)
Depression
Dyspepsia
Earache
Epilepsy
Fainting
Fevers (malarial,
   intermittent)
Gout
Hiccough
Hysteria
Insomnia
Mental fatigue
Migraine
Nausea
Nervous tension
Paralysis
Polypus (nasal)
Respiratory
   disorders
Vomiting
Whooping cough

Basil, also known as sweet basil, is called *tulsi* in India, and is extensively used in ayurvedic medicine. It is sacred to Krishna and Vishnu. It is a hairy plant, grows up to three feet in height, and has white flowers. It is a native of Asia, but is now grown in Europe, North Africa, the Seychelles, and Reunion.

The essence is a light greenish-yellow and contains linalol, which is also present in bergamot and lavender oils. It has a very pleasant, light, refreshing odour which is like a mixture of thyme, peppermint, and licorice. The taste is sweet, piercing, and slightly bitter. It gives a sweet, green top note to blends, and mixes favourably with geranium, hyssop, and bergamot. The name of basil comes from the Greek *basilicon*, meaning a 'royal' ointment or remedy.

'The smell of Basil is good for the heart . . . it taketh away sorrowfulness, which commeth of melancholy and maketh a man merry and glad.' (John Gerard).

'And away to Dr. Reason went I, who told me it was an herb of Mars, and under the Scorpion, and therefore called basilicon, and it is no marvel if it carry a kind of virulent quality with it. Being applied to the place bitten by venomous beasts, or stung by a wasp or hornet, it speedily draws the poison to it. — *Every like draws it like.* . . . It expelleth both birth and after-birth' (Nicholas Culpeper).

The Indians seem to know more about the use of basil than anyone else. The following extract is from Dr Chandrashekhar's, *Ayurveda for You*:

'The juice of leaves is fed to a person who is unconscious through snake-bite, and 1 to 2 teaspoonfuls are given at an interval of 2 to 3 hours. The juice is also applied on the whole body. It is applied in case of scorpion sting as well.

'In ordinary form, the juice of the tulsi with cinnamon, cloves, cardamom, a little sugar and milk helps a lot in common cold and influenza. It brings about perspiration, reduces fever, pain in the joints, and acts as an expectorant. Sometimes the juice of the leaf is applied all over the body in cases of malarial fever.

'A few drops of the juice poured into the ear stops earache. The juice of leaves serves as a rejuvenator if taken twice a day at the rate of one teaspoonful. It gives a flow to the complexion.

'The tulsi has been used in India from the Vedic period. At the time of epidemics and endemics it acts as a prophylactic.

'The juice of the leaves given with the juice of garlic and honey, reduces cough in a wonderful way. The juice checks vomiting; it removed intestinal worms.

'Leaf-juice is used along with honey to make medicinal preparations. In certin varieties of skin disorders like itching, ring-worm and impure blood, the juice is applied on the affected part, and also taken internally.'

Basil resembles peppermint in many ways. Its scent has the same piercing quality, but it is hotter. They are both good for fainting, indigestion, vomiting, etc. They also have a similar hot/cold quality. Mrs Grieve describes basil leaves as 'cool to the touch'; Potter mentions its 'cooling properties'; Dr Chandrashekhar describes the juice of the leaves as 'pungent, hot'. Unlike camphor, basil is predominantly yang; it is yang becoming yin while camphor is yin becoming yang. In the bath basil is uplifting and refreshing, but it also has a strong feeling on the skin, which is hot and cold at the same time, and the more you put in the water the more it stings, like a fine pinprick. It certainly comes under the Scorpion. This hot/cold effect in the bath is similar to that of peppermint oil which, however, is more definitely cold.

Drs Gatti and Cajola attribute basil with an inferior action to eucalyptus, but a superior action to thyme oil in diseases of the respiratory tract. Its affinity with peppermint and its piercing quality would seem to indicate basil as useful for sinus congestion. It is a good antiseptic, expectorant, and (neurotropic) antispasmodic and may be useful for asthma, bronchitis, and emphysema. For acute conditions it is best combined with mild expectorants. Dr Valnet recommends it for chronic colds, and Dr Chandrashekhar for colds and influenza, in combination with other warming aromatics.

Oil of basil is an excellent, indeed perhaps the best, aromatic nerve tonic. It clears the head, relieves intellectual fatigue, and gives the mind strength and clarity. It may be used in all types of nervous disorders, especially those associated with weakness, indecision, or hysteria; it is recommended by Dr Valnet for epilepsy and paralysis. Of the labiates it is one of the most pleasant oils, and is of great value in states of nervousness, anxiety, and depression. It is uplifting, clarifying, and strengthening.

Its antispasmodic action renders it an effective remedy for hiccough and whooping cough. It is a sudorific and febrifuge, and may be used for all types of fevers. In ayurvedic medicine it is combined with black pepper for malarial fever. The action of basil also resembles that of thyme. It is not such a powerful general antiseptic as thyme, and is perhaps not such a strong remedy on the physical level; it acts more on the mind and emotions. It is a more pleasant scent and a more subtle remedy, and should be used when the mind is the predominant factor in sickness relating to respiration, digestion, and the nervous system. Dr Chandrashekhar refers to it as giving a glow to the complexion; it has stimulating effect on the skin, and may be used — always in moderation — for sluggish, congested skins, or as a general tonic-refresher. The action of basil is usually enhanced by combining it with other remedies.

It has proved a useful insect repellant, particularly of mosquitoes, and has also been used for the bites of insects, snakes, and scorpions.

Basil oil is best avoided during pregnancy.

Benzoin

Latin name	*Styrax benzoin*
Family	*Styraceae*
Quality	Yang
Ruling planet	Sun
Evaporation rate	100
Odour intensity	4
Essence from	Gum

Properties
Antiseptic
Carminative
Cordial
Deodorant
Diuretic
Expectorant
Sedative
Vulnerary

Uses
Arthritis
Asthma
Bronchitis
Colic
Coughs
Gout
Laryngitis
Skin irritations
Sores
Spermatorrhoea
Wounds

The benzoin tree is cultivated in Java, Sumatra, and Thailand. The gum is not naturally produced, but forms when a deep incision is made in the trunk. This produces a slow exudation, which is collected from the tree when it has sufficiently hardened. The gum is a greyish colour with dark red streaks. It is the red parts which contain most of the aromatic material.

Benzoin, which used to be known as gum benjamin, is one of the classic ingredients of incense, and was used in ancient times in fumigations to drive away evil spirits. It is best known in the form of compound tincture of benzoin, or friar's balsam, which has done much service as an inhalation. It has a similar action to benzoic acid, its principal ingredient. It is not mentioned by many of the early herbalists, although it was known in Europe in the sixteenth century. The earliest reference I have come across is Joseph Miller:

'The tree bears large citron-like leaves, but of a paler green, and whitish underneath; the fruit is about the bigness of a nutmeg, somewhat flattish, covered with a bark like the outer shell of a walnut, but somewhat downy on the outside.

'This gum is heating and drying and . . . is of great service in opening the lungs and freeing them from their sharp, tartarous humours, which stuff them up, and by that means, it very much helps the asthma.'

A resinoid, or absolute, is produced from the gum. It is a beautiful reddish-brown colour, and has the consistency of a fatty oil. Benzoin has been imported for centuries by the Chinese, and a similar product to our modern benzoin absolute is mentioned by Li Shih-Chên:

'Liquid benzoin . . . a treacle-like oil with all the properties of the gum benzoin. It is sold in small bottles in the large medicine shops.'

Benzoin absolute has a treacly odour, resembling vanilla. Of the gums, it has one of the pleasantest odours. It blends very well with rose and sandalwood, and is an excellent fixative. A drop on the tongue produces a hot, burning sensation, although it does not actually burn. As the burning subsides it brings a pleasant warmth to the body, and a warm clarity to the head.

It is a yang sedative, and has a pronounced action on the mucous membranes. It is of particular value in disorders of the urinary and respiratory tracts. Being ruled by the sun, benzoin has a far-reaching stimulating, energising action; it seems to have the ability to 'melt away' blockages. It expectorates mucus, stimulates the flow of urine, warms and tones the heart and circulation, and expels flatulence.

Benzoin may be used with benefit in all cold conditions related to the lungs, such as colds, influenza, coughs, asthma, bronchitis. It may be used externally or in inhalations. Most of the volatile principle is eliminated via the lungs. It is also of value in cold affections of the genito-urinary system, and may be used in cystitis, albuminuria, or any conditions where there is infection or discharge, such as spermatorrhoea, gonorrhoea, and perhaps leucorrhoea.

Externally benzoin is of great value in skin conditions where there is redness, irritation, or itching, such as dermatitis; also for skin which is cracked or dry, wounds, etc. Both externally and internally is it good for cold conditions of the joints such as gout and rheumatoid arthritis. It warms the heart, both physically and metaphorically. Mme Maure says of benzoin: 'This essence creates a kind of euphoria; it interposes a padded zone between us and events.' She also recommends a blend of benzoin and cinnamon for 'exhaustion of an emotional or psychic nature'. Joseph Miller comments: 'a good cephalic, comforting the brain by its grateful smell'.

To understand the action of benzoin you only need to think of its planetary rules, the sun: heating, drying, energising, uplifting, and eventually soporific. What is there more pleasant, more euphoric, than to bathe in the warm sun?

Bergamot

Latin name	*Citrus bergamia*
Family	*Rutaceae*
Quality	Yang
Ruling planet	Sun
Evaporation rate	55
Odour intensity	4
Essence from	Fruit

Properties
Analgesic
Antidepressant
Antiseptic
Antispasmodic
Carminative
Cicatrisant
Deodorant
Digestive
Expectorant
Febrifuge
Sedative
Vermufuge
Vulnerary

Uses
Abscess (cold)
Acne
Bronchitis
Cancer (uterine)
Carbuncles
Colic
Cystitis
Depression
Diphtheria
Dyspepsia
Eczema
Fevers
Flatulence
Gall stones
Glossitis
Gonorrhoea
Halitosis
Herpes
Leucorrhoea
Nervous tension
Psoriasis
Respiratory tract
  infections
Scabies
Skin care
Stomatitis
Tonsillitis (acute)
Tuberculosis
Urinary tract
  infections
Vaginal pruritis
Varicose ulcers
Wounds, ulcers

Bergamot oil comes from the rind of a fruit which grows in Italy, and should not be confused with the herb known as bergamot, or bee balm. The latter plant is indigenous to North America, and its name arises from the fact that the scent of its leaves resembles true bergamot oil. The bergamot tree was named after the city of Bergamo in Lombardy, where the essence was first sold. The essence is extracted from the rind of the fruit, which resembles a slightly pear-shaped orange. It is one of the most widely used essences in the perfume industry, its scent and its price being superior to the other citrus oils. The scent is sweet and citrusy, but has a warm, floral quality absent in lemon and orange, and reminiscent of lavender or neroli. The taste of bergamot oil is more bitter than lemon oil, or even bitter orange oil; it is a greenish-yellow colour.

It blends well with most essences, notably jasmine, cypress, and neroli. Along with neroli and lavender it is one of the principal ingredients of the classic Eau-de-Cologne. It makes a very pleasant top note to almost any blend, and is a freshing and relaxing bath oil.

Li Shih-chên says:

> 'The fruits of all the different species and varieties [of citrus] are considered by the Chinese to be cooling. If eaten in excess they are thought to increase the "phlegm", and this is probably not advantageous to the health. The sweet varieties increase bronchial secretion, and the sour promote expectoration. They all quench thirst, and are stomachic and carminative.'

He states that the dried peel of citrus is stomachic, carminative, stimulant, tonic, antiphlogistic, and deodorant. Bergamots do not grow in China, but there are several varieties of oranges, which are very popular in Chinese medicine. Orange peel is recommended for marasmus in children, pin worms, and breast cancer.

Rovesti recommends bergamot oil for cancer of the uterus, not as a curative agent, but apparently to minimise many of the symptoms and side-effects. Citrus oils in general are known to be slightly irritating, and in very large amounts have produced experimental tumours in mice. The tumours were benign, and were not easy to produce, especially with bergamot oil. Nevertheless some association appears to exist between tumours and citrus oils, and it may well be a homoeopathic one; what a large dose will produce, a very small dose will cure.

Bergamot oil has been used in Italian folk medicine for many years, primarily for fevers and worms. Being indigenous to Italy

189

bergamots do not figure in the traditional medicine of other countries. In 1960 Paolo Rovesti published an article entitled 'L'aromaterapia dell'essenza di Bergamotta' which has been my main source of information.

Used in douches and hip baths bergamot oil has proved successful in gonococcal infections, leucorrhoea, and vaginal pruritis. In cancer of the uterus is minimises local infection, purulent secretions, and irritation of the genitalia. It has a wide application as an antiseptic, and is effective against gonococcus, staphylococcus, coli, meningococcus, vibrio Nasik, diphtheria bacillus, and many more. It is of particular value in infections of the mouth, skin, respiratory and urinary tracts, and is indicated in diphtheria, tonsillitis, and most types of sore throat.

Bergamot oil has a slightly irritating effect on the skin in high concentrations but, if used in moderation (1% or less), it has the reverse effect. It has been found useful in eczema, psoriasis, and acne, and is a good antiseptic and healing agent in indolent wounds and ulcers. It has also been used in seborrhoea of the skin and scalp, and acts as a parasiticide in scabies. It is an effective deodorising agent.

It is also effective against tuberculous bacilli, and is indicated in all types of respiratory tract infections, especially bronchitis; in this respect it is most effective when mixed with lemon oil. As a disinfectant of oral bacteria it helps to eliminate bad breath. Its antiseptic action is strongly indicated in cystitis and urinary tract infections. Bergamot is useful in all types of fever including those of the intermittent, malarial type. Its action on the digestive tract is antispasmodic, carminative, digestive, and it is one of the many aromatic remedies for colic, flatulence, and indigestion.

As a nerve sedative it is valuable for depression and states of anxiety, and its pleasant odour makes it as useful as rose or sandalwood in this capacity. Unlike them it has a light, refreshing odour, and has a greater uplifting, lightening quality. Bergamot oil is used to flavour Earl Grey tea.

Bergamot oil has the effect of increasing the photosensitivity of the skin, which therefore tans more readily. *However, it must never be used neat on the skin in the presence of sunlight or ultra-violet light.* Even when diluted in a vegetable oil, remember that it will not protect our skin from the burning rays of the sun!

Black Pepper

Latin name	*Piper nigrum*
Family	*Piperaceae*
Quality	Yang
Ruling planet	Mars
Evaporation rate	60
Odour intensity	7
Essence from	Fruit (known as peppercorns)

Properties
Analgesic
Antiseptic
Antispasmodic
Antitoxic
Aphrodisiac
Carminative
Digestive
Diuretic
Febrifuge
Laxative
Rubefacient
Stimulant
Stomachic
Tonic (especially
   of the spleen)

Uses
Catarrh
Cholera
Cold
Colic
Constipation
Cough
Diarrhoea
Dysentery
Dyspepsia
Dysuria
Fevers
Flatulence
Heartburn
Influenza
Loss of appetite

Nausea
Quinsy
Toothache
Vertigo
Vomiting

Black peppers are cultivated in Malabar, Java, Sumatra, and Penang. The plant grows naturally to a height of twenty feet or more, but is restricted to twelve feet for commerical purposes. Black peppercorns are the sun-dried red berries, which are picked before they are ripe. White peppercorns are from the same plant but the berries are not picked until they are fully ripe, and the pericarp (outer layer) is removed before drying.

Our word pepper originates from the Latin *piper* which in turn comes from the Sanskrit *pippali*. Pepper, like cinnamon and cloves, is one of the oldest known spices, and was being used in India over 4,000 years ago. It was also extensively used in ancient Greece and Rome and 3,000 years ago had already become an important article of commerce.

Oil of black pepper is a light amber colour, and smells very like clove oil, but has a more pleasant, more refined scent. It will blend with sandalwood and frankincense. Being under Mars it has a very hot quality, and the taste is moderately bitter.

'This is called pepper. It is hot and dry in the fourth degree. There be three manner of peppers, black, white, and long pepper. . . . But of all the peppers the black is the best and the most wholesome. Take pepper and put it into thy nostrils and it will make thee to sneeze . . . And it is for the pose [catarrh] that is taken of cold . . . Also, black pepper hath virtue of loosing, comforting, and of drawing. It cleanseth the spiritual members of cold, phlegm, and vicous-humours, and best when the powder of it is eaten with figs, for it hath a great strength of heating and of comforting the stomach and provoking appetite, but to sanguine and choleric persons it is not good to use pepper . . .' (Banckes's *Herbal*).

'All the peppers are under the dominion of Mars, and of temperature hot and dry, almost to the fourth degree; but the white is the hottest. It comforts and warms a cold stomach, consumes crude and moist humours, and stirs up the appetite. It dissolves wind in the stomach or bowels, provokes urine, helps the cough, and other diseases of the breast, and is an ingredient in the great antidotes . . . being used for agues, to warm the stomach before the coming of the fit. All are used against the quinsy, being mixed with honey and taken inwardly and applied outwardly, to disperse the kernels in the throat, and other places' (Nicholas Culpeper).

'Pepper is heating and drying, expelling wind, and of great use against coldness and windiness of the stomach, and the colic; it strengthens the nerves and head, and helps the sight; outwardly it is good for the tooth-ache, and for cold affections of the nerves, and pains in the limbs' (Joseph Miller).

'Carminative, warming, and eliminative properties are ascribed to the drug, and it is administered in cholera, dysentery, vomiting, summer diarrhoea, and dysuria. It is said to correct fish flesh, shell-fish, and mushroom poisoning . . . Pepper essence is stomachic, peptic, stimulant, and tonic to the spleen' (Li Shih-Chên).

'Aromatic, stimulant, carminative; is said to possess febrifuge properties. Its action as a stimulant is specially evident on the mucous membrane of the rectum, and so is good for constipation, also on the urinary organs; externally it is a rubefacient, useful in relaxed conditions of the rectum when prolapsed; sometimes used in place of cubebs for gonorrhoea; given in combination with aperients to facilitate their action, and to prevent griping' (Mrs Grieve). [cubeb: an aromatic berry from Java]

Dr Chandrashekhar recommends black pepper for dyspepsia, colic, cough, piles, urinary disorders, diseases of the chest, and colds. In rural areas of India powdered black pepper is given as an inhalation in cases of fainting and hysteria. Wren recommends pepper for flatulence, congestive chills, and intermittent fevers. Marguerite Maury tells us that 'in Greece the plant was used against intermittent fever which was in actual fact a mild form of Mediterranean malaria'. Culpeper also recommends pepper for 'agues, to warm the stomach before the coming of the fit'. Ague is intermittent fever. Mme Maury continues: 'experience has taught us that the essential oil of pepper exerts a great influence on the muscular tonus. We often use it in the case of muscular atonia.'

In homoeopathic practice black pepper is used for difficulty in concentrating, heavy headache with aching eyeballs, nosebleed, flatulence, colic, cough with pain in the chest, palpitation, cardiac pain, burning or difficult urination, and a sad, apprehensive state of mind.

Black pepper oil is hot, warming, very yang. Its principal areas of action are the urinary, respiratory, and digestive system. It is a stimulating oil, and inevitably has something of a cephalic quality, operating on the mind. It stimulates urination and digestion, and is a stimulating aphrodisiac. It has a pronounced stimulating action of the digestive tract, hence its use in atonic dyspepsia, constipation, flatulence, loss of appetite, etc. It appears to restore tone to lax smooth musculatures — prolapsed colon, uterus, etc.

Black pepper is indicated whenever there is an excess of cold or water. If there is an excess of heat it should only be used in small quantities, diluted to less than 1% (as in aromatic waters). It is a good remedy for acute conditions, and also for chronic ones, but here it is best combined with other essences.

As a warming essence black pepper is, like all hot spices, good for colds and influenza; it is a good remedy for fevers, especially of the intermittent type. It stimulates the circulation, is a spleen tonic, and acts as an antitoxic agent, especially with regard to certain types of food poisoning, as the quotation from Li Shih-Chên indicated. Culpeper's comment that 'it is an ingredient in all the great antidotes' refers to the classical use of certain aromatics to antidote attempted poisoning.

Externally it is rubefacient and gently analgesic, especially good for muscular aches and pains and for sharp pain such as toothache or angina. As a rubefacient and stimulant it is sometimes successful in cases of rhematoid arthritis or paralysis. As a very yang remedy it is indicated where there is extreme cold, physical or emotional.

Camomile

Latin name	*Anthemis nobilis*
	Matricaria chamomilla
Family	*Compositae*
Quality	Yin
Ruling planet	Moon
Evaporation rate	47
Odour intensity	9
Essence from	Flowers

Properties	**Uses**	
Analgesic	Allergies	Hysteria
Anticonvulsive	Anaemia	Insomnia
Antidepressant	Boils	Irritability
Antiphlogistic	Burns	Jaundice
Antiseptic	Colic	Menopausal
Antispasmodic	Colitis	problems
Carminative	Conjunctivitis	Menorrhagia
Cholagogue	Convulsions	Migraine
Cicatrisant	Depression	Nephritis
Digestive	Dermatitis	Neuralgia
Diuretic	Diarrhoea	Rheumatism
Emmenagogue	Dysmenorrhoea	Stones (urinary)
Febrifuge	Dyspepsia	Teething pains
Hepatic	Earache	Toothache
Nervine	Fevers	Ulcers (peptic)
Sedative	Flatulence	Urticaria
Splenetic	Gastalgia	Vaginitis
Stomachic	Gastritis	Vertigo
Sudorific	Gingivitis	Vomiting
Tonic	Headache	Vulvar pruritis
		Wounds

Properties

Vasoconstrictor
  (local)
Vermifuge
Vulnerary

Known to the Saxons as *maythen*, camomile is one of the oldest known English medicinal herbs. Along with lavender and peppermint it is one of the principal oil-producing herbs grown in this country. The fragrance of camomile flowers has often been likened to that of apples, and it was called *kamai melon* (ground-apple) by the Greeks, which gave rise to the English name. Camomile used to be regarded as the 'plant's physician', and was thought to keep other plants in good health. Camomiles belong to the daisy family, and strongly resemble common daisies. When walked on their fragrance becomes noticeable, and they were often used as 'strewing herbs' in the Middle Ages, and purposely planted along garden paths.

There are a number of species of camomile growing in Europe, North Africa, and the temperate region of Asia. Four species can be found growing in the wild in England, and of these only one is commonly used in medicine; this is *Anthemis nobilis*, also known as Roman camomile. It grows to about a foot in height, has fine, feathery leaves, and the flower consists of a yellow centre covered with tiny white petals. *Matricaria chamomilla*, which is found in the more eastern parts of Europe, is similar in appearance except that it has a smaller flower head and fewer petals. It is the type most commonly used as camomile tea, and is known as German camomile.

Interest in camomiles has recently been revived because of the discovery that they contain azulene. When isolated this substance takes the form of intensely blue crystals. It has been found to be an excellent anti-inflammatory agent, and only very small quantities need to be used. It is now being used in a growing number of pharmaceutical preparations and toiletries. Azulene is not present in the fresh flower, but is formed when the essential oil is distilled. It may also be formed when the flowers are dried.

Roman camomiles contain about 1% of essential oil, and the German flowers contain about 0.25%. Azulene is present in both oils, but is more predominant in German camomile oil. The

196

colour of the oils varies from the very light blue of Roman camomile to the deep blue of the German oil. The odour of the Roman oil is light, refreshing, and reminiscent of apples, and the taste is bitter but relatively pleasant. Camomile oil blends well with rose, geranium, and lavender and makes a light and relaxing bath oil.

'This oil is called camomile. The virtue of this herb is thus. If it be drunken with wine, it will break the stone. Also, it destroyeth the yellow evil. It helpeth the aching and the disease of the liver. If it be strained, it helpeth and assuageth the sores in a man's mouth. It is good for the aching of a man's head and for the megrim.' (Banckes's *Herbal*).

'It hath floures wonderfully shynynge yellow and resemblynge the appell of an eye . . . the herbe may be called in English, golden floure. It will restore a man to hys color shortly yf a man after the longe use of the bathe drynke of it after he is come for the oute of the bath' (William Turner).

'A decoction made of camomile, taketh away all pains and stitches in the side: the flowers of camomile beaten and made into balls with oil, drive away all sorts of agues, if the part grieved be anointed with that oil, taken from the flowers, from the crown of the head to the sole of the foot, and afterward lay to sweat in bed, and he sweats well; this is Nechessor, an Egyptian's medicine.

'It is profitable for all sorts of agues that come either from phlegm, or melancholy, or from an inflammation of the bowels, being applied when the humours causing them shall be concocted: and there is nothing more profitable to the sides and region of the liver and spleen than it . . . it easeth all the pains of the colic and stone, and all pains and torments of the belly, and gently provoketh urine. The flowers boiled in posset-drink provoke sweat, and help to expel all colds, aches and pains whatsoever: it is an excellent help to bring down women's courses. Syrup made of the juice of camomile, with the flowers in white wine, is a remedy against the jaundice and dropsy.

'The oil made of the flowers of camomile is much used against all hard swellings, pains or aches, shrinking of the sinews, cramps or pains in the joints, or any other part of the body. Being used in clysters, it helps to dissolve the wind and pains in the belly; anointed also, it helpeth pains and stitches in the sides.

'Also this is certain, that it most wonderfully breaks the stone; some take it in syrup or decoction, others inject the juice of it into the bladder with a syringe . . . That it is excellent for the stone appears in this which I have seen tried, viz; that a stone that hath been taken out of the body of a man, being wrapped in camomile, will in time dissolve, and in a little time too' (Nicholas Culpeper)

Joseph Miller describes Roman camomile as 'a plant of many virtues. being stomachic, hepatic, nervine, emollient and carminative'. He recommends it for colic, jaundice, urinary stones, agues, and in fomentations for inflammations and tumours. William Whitla describes it as an aromatic stimulant, and stomachic bitter, 'improving the appetite and aiding digestion by increasing the vascularity of the mucous membrane. Its chief use is in atonic dyspepsia.' He refers to the essential oil as stimulant and antispasmodic, and states that it diminishes reflex excitability. Mrs Grieve refers to camomile as tonic, stomachic, anodyne, and antispasmodic. She commends it as a remedy for hysterical and nervous affections in women, and as an emmenagogue. She writes: 'It has a wonderfully soothing, sedative, and absolutely harmless effect.'

Camomile essence has a relatively low toxicity, and has been an official preparation for over 250 years. It is strongly indicated in any inflammatory condition, whether internal or external, hence its use in burns, conjunctivitis, dermatitis, gastritis, diarrhoea, colitis, nephritis, and so on. It is a mile antispasmodic and diuretic, and may also be useful in asthma, bronchitis, and cystitis. It is a very good remedy for digestive disorders, and is especially good for peptic ulcers, because of its antiphlogistic and vulnerary properties, and because of its general sedative action. In some cases it will relieve vomiting due to gastritis or blood poisoning when all other remedies fail. In homoeopathic practice camomile is indicated in foul belching, the rising of acid into the mouth, or bilious vomiting.

Camomile is often indicated when there is aching or pains generally, whether in the muscles, bones, or organs. In particular we may mention earache, headache, migraine, low backache, aching of the liver or spleen, abdominal aches or pains, period pains, rheumatic pains, toothache, teething pains of infants, and facial neuralgia. Camomile is a good remedy for urinary stones, and is strongly indicated when there is inflammation of the renal pelvis or ureter due to the presence of stones. A massage oil made with camomile essence is good for muscular aches due to sporting activities, or excessive heat in the muscles.

Dr Valnet cites camomile oil as a stimulant of leucocytosis and as being good for engorgement of the spleen; Culpeper mentions that it is 'excellent for the spleen'. It is therefore useful in almost any type of infection (as are other leucocytosis-stimulating essences) especially when it is associated with a low resistance and repeated susceptibility to infection. Camomile oil is also very good for the liver. Dr Valnet mentions its use in anaemia and engorgement of the liver and Culpeper recommends it for jaundice. Its anti-inflammatory action may be useful in cholecystitis.

Camomile is good for many female disorders, including scanty menstruation, painful or irregular periods, excessive loss of blood during periods, uterine haemorrhages, vaginitis, vulvar itching, and menopausal problems. It is especially indicated when these are associated with nervous disorders. Its efficacy in female disorders gave rise to the German name which translated means 'mother herb'.

Camomile has a pronounced effect on the mind and the nervous system. Culpeper mentions that it comforts both the head and the brain, and it has been traditionally used for hysterical and nervous affections. It is both sedative and antidepressant. It is useful for mental, as well as physical, aches and pains, and is indicated when there is restlessness, nervous irritability, or impatience. Associated with its action on the liver is its usefulness in states of anger, the choleric or livid humour of the old herbalists (this quality is also apparent in rose, another antiphlogistic oil). Camomile is indicated when there is over-sensitiveness, either physical or emotional, and the oil has been shown to be anti-allergic as well as antiphlogistic.

Oil of camomile is a well-known remedy for children's ailments, primarily due to its low toxicity, and its anti-inflammatory and sedative action. It is indicated in peevishness, convulsions, temper tantrums, over-sensitivity, colic, diarrhoea, gastric spasms, asthma, teething pains, earaches, and other disorders where there is inflammation or pain.[1]

Camomile was used by the ancient Egyptians for agues (intermittent fevers) and has been used in a similar way by herbalists ever since. In a Polish study (1966) camomile oil was shown to lower the body temperature of rats by $3 - 3.5°$. Several herbalists have recommended the use of camomile for tumours, notably, Joseph Miller. Camomile oil lowers high blood urea in rats due to experimental glomeronephritis.

Applied to the skin camomile oil is analgesic, antiphlogistic, cicatrisant, and antiseptic. Its uses as an analgesic have already been enumerated. Its combination of properties make it an excellent remedy for burns, and it may be used on inflamed wounds, ulcers, or boils. It is indicated in any type of skin inflammation, and is good for dermatitis, acne, or hypersensitive skin; its antiphlogistic action is synonymous with constriction of the blood capillaries. It is also good for dry skin, especially when there is redness or sensitivity. As an anti-allergic agent camomile is useful for skin eruptions due to allergies, and it is very good for urticaria. It is often used in herbal shampoos, and is said to lighten the hair.

It should always be remembered that German camomile, due to its higher azulene content, is a more potent remedy for inflammatory conditions than Roman camomile.

1 For infants always use internally, and diluted.

Camphor

Latin name	Cinnamomum camphora
Family	Lauraceae
Quality	Yin
Ruling planet	Saturn
Evaporation rate	?
Odour intensity	5
Essence from	Wood

Properties
Analgesic
Anthelmintic
Antidepressant
Antiseptic
Antispasmodic
Carminative
Diuretic
Febrifuge
Hypertensive
Laxative
Rubefacient
Sedative
Stimulant (of circu-
    lation, digestion,
    heart and
    respiration)
Sudorific
Vaso-constrictor
    (systemic)
Vulnerary

Uses
Acne
Bronchitis
Bruises
Burns
Cholera
Colds
Colic
Constipation
Debility
Depression
Diarrhoea
Fevers
Flatulence
Gout
Heart failure
Hypotension
Hysteria
Inflammatory
    affections
Insomnia

Nervous tension
Pneumonia
Retention of urine
Rheumatism
Shock
Skin care
Sprains
Toothache
Tuberculosis
Ulcers
Vomiting
Wounds

Camphor is obtained from very large, hardy trees indigenous to

Formosa, China, and Japan, and has been successfully
cultivated in other sub-tropical countries such as India, Ceylon,
and Madagascar. The tree, an evergreen, grows slowly and may
reach up to 100 feet in height, with a trunk between eight and
ten feet in diameter. The trunk usually runs straight up for
twenty to thirty feet before it branches out. The leaves are small,
elliptical, and slightly serrated. The flowers are white, small,
and clustered; the fruits are dark-red berries.

Camphor is present in every part of the tree, but takes many
years to form, and trees are not touched until they are fifty years
old. In the trunk it is present in masses twelve to eighteen inches
long. It is extracted from the branches by chipping the wood,
and then boiling it in water. The camphor then rises to the surface, and becomes solid as the water cools. The oil is extracted
by steam distillation. It is clear, and has a pungent scent similar
to that of eucalyptus.

Camphor does not appear in English herbals until the late
seventeenth century. Joseph Miller writes:

> 'Camphire consists of hot subtile parts, resists
> putrefaction and malignant distempers, is good in
> putrid, pestilential fevers attended with delirium, or
> light-headedness. Outwardly used, it is of great service
> in all sorts of inflammations, St. Anthony's Fire,
> ophthalmia, burns and scalds. It is made use of as a
> corrector of cantharides; some people hang it in a silk
> bag, about the neck to cure agues.'

There appears to be some confusion as to whether camphor is
basically heating or cooling. Li Shih-Chên writes that camphor
has 'a strong terebinthinate odour, and a warm, bitter, aromatic
taste, with a somewhat cooling after taste'. Mrs Grieve calls it
'cold to the touch' and Dr Chandrashekhar 'cold in action'.
This is difficult to reconcile with Joseph Miller's comments, and
with the fact that camphor is also used as a rubefacient and is a
stimulant of the heart and circulation. Christian Samuel
Hahnemann, the father of modern homoeopathy, throws considerable light on the matter:

> 'The action of this substance is very puzzling and dif-
> ficult of investigation, even in the healthy organism
> because its action, more frequently than with any

other remedy, alternates and becomes intermixed with the vital reactions of the organism. On this account it is often difficult to determine what belongs to the vital reactions of the body and what to the alternating effects due to the primary action of the camphor.'

While puzzling over the action of camphor, I was reminded that yin and yang are not two opposing, fixed objects. Nor only is one always contained within the other, but there is a constant transformation from one into the other. As something becomes more and more yin it eventually reaches a stage of instability, since nothing can become totally yin, and it then changes to predominantly yang.

The action of camphor is akin to yin changing into yang, and it shows both qualities quite strongly. At first sight it always appears to me as yin. Its action on the skin is cooling, and it is a useful anti-inflammatory agent. Everyone has felt how something very cold burns as if it were hot: the action of a cold agent can produce a strong reaction of heat, just as a cold wind on the face stimulates the circulation. This, in many ways, represents the action of camphor. From Hahnemann's comments (which are based on considerable experience) we can see that its action depends, perhaps more than any other essence, on the state of the person it is applied to. If their state at the time is very yin this will precipitate the yang reaction; if they are more yang, the action of camphor may remain predominantly yin.

Being a powerful remedy it is of great use in certain serious conditons. It is a strong heart stimulant, and may be given in cases of heart failure, whether due to extreme shock, cardiac disease, or as a result of infectious fevers, such as typhoid and pneumonia. It has other uses for pneumonia, being active against the pneumococcus bacteria, and also being a stimulant of the circulation. In homoeopathy camphor is especially indicated in coldness of the whole body (this will produce a strong yang reaction). Any condition where there is coldness — the common cold, a cold stomach, influenza, a fever accompanied by a feeling of coldness — indicates the use of camphor.

Because of its almost dual action camphor is also useful where there is a state of excess yang: a burning fever, rheumatic inflammation, a skin burn, or any other kind of inflammation. It is of considerable use in dressings for indolent wounds and ulcers, and as an ingredient in external applications for skins of the oily, acne type. Applied externally camphor numbs the peripheral nerve endings.

Its effect on the digestive system is antispasmodic, carminative, laxative, and it stimulates the flow of digestive juices. It is useful, not only in constipation, but also in diarrhoea, vomiting, colic, flatulence, and cholera. Camphor is best kept in reserve for the more serious alimentary complaints, such as acute diarrhoea. It should not be habitually used as a laxative.

Camphor oil stimulates the heart and respiration, and raises low blood pressure. It is indicated when these functions are weakened. This may occur in serious states of depression, after an operation, and during or after serious illness such as cholera or tuberculosis. Camphor effectively inhibits mycobacterium tuberculosis. It is a useful ingredient of inhalations for coughs, colds, influenza, bronchitis, tuberculosis, and difficulty of breathing. It relieves irritation of the sexual organs, and is a powerful diuretic. It is said by some to be an aphrodisiac, and by others to be the opposite. The latter quality seems more likely.

It appears that camphor has a balancing effect on yin and yang. Hence its usefulness in conditions where this balance is either suddenly or seriously upset: shock, heart failure, hysteria, excess of heat or cold, infection. This balancing effect is also apparent in its effect on the nervous system. It stimulates languid depression, and sedates hysteria; it is of use in most psychosomatic or nervous diseases. Camphor will often produce results where milder remedies are insufficiently effective, or when a gentle shock is required in order to produce some reaction from a chronically sick body.

Remember that 100-foot high tree, and how long it took to grow and produce its camphor. Camphor oil is not expensive, but it should be used wisely, and only when needed.

Cardamon

Latin name	*Elettaria cardamomum*
Family	Zingiberaceae
Quality	Yang
Ruling planet	Mercury
Evaporation rate	68
Odour intensity	9
Essence from	Seeds

Properties
Antiseptic
Antispasmodic
Aphrodisiac
Carminative
Cephalic
Digestive
Diuretic
Stomachic
Tonic

Uses
Colic
Cough
Debility
Dyspepsia
Flatulence
Halitosis
Headache
Loss of appetite
Nausea
Pyrosis
Vomiting
Mental fatigue

The cardamon (or, if you prefer, -mom) plant flourishes in southern India and Ceylon, and several other species are to be found in China and Indo-China. In India it grows in forests 2,500 to 5,000 feet above sea-level in North Canara, Coorgi, and Wynaad, where it is also largely cultivated. It has a large, fleshy rhizome, similar to that of ginger, to which it is botanically related. Its leaves are like green silky blades between one foot and two and a half feet long, and its small flowers are usually yellowish, with a violet lip. The fruits are ovoid, about half an inch long, and turn grey when ripe. They contain three sections, each with two rows of small, reddish-brown seeds.

Cardamon oil is clear, relatively expensive, and has a very agreeable, warm, sweet, spicy scent. Its use is comparatively recent, although it may have been distilled locally in India for several centuries. It is still current in most pharmacopoeias, as a flavouring agent, and sometimes also as a carminative. Joseph Miller writes:

> 'The true amomum is warming and comforting, strengthens the stomach, helps digestion, expels wind, and is good against the collick and cold disorders of the stomach and bowels, as also against the bitings of venomous creatures; it is useful to promote urine and the catamenia.'

It is moderately yang, gently warming, and is a general tonic. Its primary action is on the digestion system. In this it compares favourably with peppermint oil, and together they form a powerful alimentary team. Cardamon is sometimes used as a corrective in laxatives, and is probably underestimated for its value in colic. My wife can vouch for it as bringing relief in pregnancy nausea. Like peppermint it will relieve nausea, but does not prevent vomiting if you really need to vomit. After vomiting it speedily comforts and warms the stomach, and helps to put the head and palate back in place. As well as correcting indigestion it is an effective remedy for pyrosis, or heartburn, although persistent heartburn may be a symptom of a more serious problem, such as hiatus hernia. It also helps to correct unnatural gastric fermentation, which is often the cause of foul breath (halitosis). Dr Chandrashekhar recommends cardamon for coughs, difficulty in passing urine, and indigestion and gas caused by eating an excessive quantity of bananas!

Although it primarily affects the digestive system, cardamon oil does have other uses. Most people find its odour extremely pleasant, and it is my own experience that it has a distinct uplifting, lightening effect, helping to clear the mind of noise and confusion. It is what Culpeper would have called cephalic, and Mrs Grieve mentions its use in disorders of the head. It may not have a physiological effect on the nervous system, but it certainly has a psychological effect, and is especially good for digestive problems of nervous origin. Related to this is its tonic and aphrodisiac effect. Cardamon is often used in Eastern aphrodisiacs, although one cannot be certain whether or not there is any physiological effect. As a general tonic and mild stimulant it may be of service in any condition where there is general debility, and more particularly when this is related to a weak digestion. It has also been used in China for pulmonary disease and for intermittent fever. It may be of use here, but one feels that it would have a relatively weak effect if used alone. Cardamon oil blends well with most other essences although, having a high odour intensity, it makes its presence known very rapidly. It makes an excellent bath oil, light, refreshing and stimulating.

Cedarwood

Latin name	*Juniperus virginiana*
Family	*Coniferae*
Quality	Yang
Ruling planet	Uranus
Evaporation rate	97
Odour intensity	4
Essence from	Wood

Properties
Antiseptic
Astringent
Diuretic
Expectorant
Sedative

Uses
Acne
Bronchitis
Cancer?
Catarrh
Cystitis
Dysuria
Gonorrhoea
Pyelitis
Respiratory affections
Skin diseases
Urinary tract disorders

'Thy lips, O my spouse, drop as the honeycomb:
honey and milk are under thy tongue; and the smell
of thy garments is like the smell of Lebanon'
(*Song of Solomon*).

Unfortunately the Lebanon cedar (*Cedrus libani*) which was the one used by the ancients, no longer grows as abundantly as it once did. There used to be great forests of these enormous trees, but over the centuries they have been considerably reduced by the great demand for cedarwood furniture. The wood was used in building temples and palaces in the Middle East, and vast quantities were used to build Solomon's great temple in Jerusalem. Today only a few hundred trees survive.

Cedarwood oil was possibly the first essential oil to be extracted from a plant, and was used by the Egyptians in the mummification process. They also valued it highly as an ingredient for cosmetics, and impregnated papyrus leaves with it to protect them from insects. They used the wood to make jewellery, furniture, and ships, and used nothing else for their coffins. They valued cedarwood so highly that the Lebanon area was incorporated into the Egyptian empire, in order to ensure a regular supply.

There are two commercial oils which are known by the name of cedarwood. The oil from *Cedrus atlantica*, which is a true cedar, is known as Atlas cedarwood oil, and comes from Morocco. The other oils comes from *Juniperus virginiana*, a coniferous tree which grows in North America. This is known as the red cedar, and is closely related to the yellow cedar (*Thuja occidentalis* from the leaves of which thuja oil is obtained.

The red cedar is used for making pencils, and it is difficult to smell the essence without thinking of pencils! The oils is clear and relatively viscid, like sandalwood oil; it blends well with rose, juniper, and cypress, and is used as a fixative in perfumes. Therapeutically it resembles sandalwood to some degree; it has an equally bland fragrance but is hotter and more toxic. The taste is very slightly bitter.

Red cedarwood oil acts primarily on the skin, and the respiratory and genito-urinary tracts. It is said to be at least as good as sandalwood for mucous-like discharges and gonorrhoea. Its precise antiseptic effects are unknown. It should be given when there is pain, burning, or difficulty in urinating, and is a valuable remedy for cystitis. It is also indicated in pyelitis and hyperaemia of the kidneys.

Like sandalwood oil it has a pronounced effect on mucous membranes, and is good in all catarrhal conditions, especially coughs and bronchitis. It may be used with other essences in inhalations for all types of respiratory complaints. Like sandalwood it also has a sedative effect, and may be used in conditions associated with anxiety and nervous tension; it is generally more useful for chronic complaints than acute ones.

Cedarwood has a pronounced effect on the skin, and is of value in all types of skin eruptions. Its action is sedative, astringent, antiseptic, and it relieves itching. It is very good for acne, oily skin, and seborrhoea of the scalp (oily hair, dandruff) and has been recommended for traumatic alopecia. It may also be of value in more serious conditions such as eczema, dermatitis, and psoriasis. In high concentrations it will irritate the skin.

It is a very good insect repellent, and is effective against a variety of fauna including mosquitoes, moths, woodworms, leeches, and rats! Since it has been shown to inhibit the mitosis[1] of tumour cells, it may be of value in cancer therapy. This action is due to its oily consistency, and is shared by turpentine and various fatty acids. Atlas cedarwood oil probably has a very similar action to that of red cedarwood. Its use has been mentioned in connection with bronchitis, gonorrhoea, urinary and respiratory infections, phthisis, and tuberculosis.

1 mitosis — cell division.

Clary Sage

Latin name	Salvia sclarea
Family	Labiatae
Quality	Yang
Ruling planet	Mercury
Evaporation rate	82
Odour intensity	5
Essence from	Herb

Properties
Anticonvulsive
Antidepressant
Antiphlogistic
Antiseptic
Antispasmodic
Aphrodisiac
Astringent
Carminative
Deodorant
Digestive
Emmenagogue
Hypotensive
Nervine
Sedative
Stomachic
Tonic
Uterine

Uses
Amenorrhoea
Boils
Colic
Convulsions
Depression
Dysmenorrhoea
Dyspepsia
Flatulence
Frigidity
Hypertension
Hysteria
Impotence
Kidney disorders
Leucorrhoea
Neurasthenia
Ophthalmia
Skin care
Throat infections
Ulcers
Whooping cough

Clary sage is similar in appearance to common sage, although its blue flowers are slightly smaller. It has broad, wrinkled leaves which are green with a hint of purple. The flower-buds are enclosed by pointed green bracts, which are sometimes streaked with purple. Both leaves and bracts are highly aromatic. The name clary stems from the Latin *sclarea* which derives from *clarus*, meaning clear. One of the synonyms for clary is 'clear eye'. This came about due to the use of a mucilage made from the seeds for clearing the eyes of foreign bodies. The name clary, however, does not actually derive from 'clear eye', as has been suggested; in fact it may have been the other way round.

This plant was known and used by the ancients, and is a native of Syria, Italy, France, and Switzerland. It is cultivated for essential oil production in France and the USSR. Mrs Grieve states that it was introduced to England in 1562. It was used in Europe in the Middle Ages, but has not been used much for medicinal purposes in recent years. In this context it has been overshadowed by common sage, rather as myrrh has overshadowed frankincense.

In Germany clary is known as *muskateller salbei*, or muscatel sage. Apparently it was originally used by German wine makers to simulate true muscatel wine. The first time I used clary sage oil was when giving a massage, and both myself and the patient became rather intoxicated. At first I was not sure if it was the clary oil, but every time I have taken it, or inhaled it for a time, it has had a similar effect. It slows one down, brings on a feeling of euphoria, and makes concentration difficult. It is much more like the effect of cannabis than alcohol. I was still not sure if this was generally true of clary, or just a subjective experience, until I came across the following passages in *A Modern Herbal*:

> 'Waller (1822) states it was also employed in this country as a substitute for Hops, for sophisticating beer, communicating considerable bitterness and intoxicating property, which produced an effect of insane exhilaration of spirits, succeeded by severe headache.
>
> 'Lobel says: "Some brewers of Ale and Beere doe put it into their drinke to make it more heady, fit to please drunkards, who thereby, according to their several dispositions, become either dread drunke, or foolish drunke, of madde drunke." '

I have never combined clary oil with alcohol, but on its own it does not produce headaches. Nicholas Culpeper comments:

'The leaves used with vinegar, either by itself or with a little honey, doth help boils, felons, and the hot inflammations that are gathered by their pains, if applied before it be grown too great . . . The seeds or leaves taken in wine provoketh to venery. It is of much use both for men and women that have weak backs, and helpeth to strengthen the reins . . . The juice of the herb put into ale or beer, and then drunk, bringeth down women's courses and expelleth the after-birth.'

'Clary is accounted to be of a warming and drying nature; infused in wine it comforts a cold windy stomach.

It is particularly commended to strengthen the reins, to help a fluor albus, and invigorate a cold, relaxed womb' (Joseph Miller).

'In Jamaica, where the plant is found, it was much in use among the negroes, who considered it cooling and cleansing for ulcers, and also used it for inflammations of the eyes. A decoction of the leaves boild in coco-nut oil was used by them to cure the stings of scorpions. Clary and a Jamaican species of Vervain form two of the ingredients of an aromatic warm bath sometimes prescribed there with benefit' (Mrs Grieve).

The essential oil is clear, and has a sweet, nutty scent, only slightly reminiscent of common sage oil, with a much more pleasant, almost floral quality. It has a quite unique appeal, and is one of my favourite scents. The taste is warm, and moderately bitter. Clary blends well with oils of juniper, lavender, and sandalwood; it is often used as a fixative in perfumes. A clary sage bath is warming and very relaxing.

Clary sage is a good oil to use as a general tonic, like juniper and common sage. Its tonic effects apply particularly to the nerves, stomach, kidneys, and uterus. Its effect on the nervous system is sedative, anticonvulsive, and tonic. It also appears to produce a mild form of euphoric intoxication, although this is not directly related to its toxicity, since very small doses are effective. Although clary is less toxic than common sage, very large doses should not be taken to induce intoxication; the result will be poisoning and a severe headache, rather than euphoria. The aphrodisiac quality of clary is intimately related to its euphoria-producing property.

As a nerve tonic clary is very good for nervous, weak, fearful types, and may be used in convalescence. It is useful in all types of debility, whether physical, mental, nervous, or sexual. As a euphoric-tonic-sedative it is useful in nervous depression and 'weakness of spirit'; it is usually effective in cases of the depression which often accompanies acute physical illness, such as influenza. and also in cases of post-natal depression.

According to Caujolle and Franck (1945) clary sage oil produced an increse in blood pressure when introduced by intravenous injection to dogs. This effect persisted for almost an hour, and appeared to be due to a stimulation of adrenalin secretion, rather than of the nerves. Shipochliev (1968) found that clary sage oil, given intravenously to experimental animals, produced a decrease in blood pressure In the first case the dose was about 1 cc per kilo of body weight, and in the second case it was 5 – 10 mg per kilo of body weight, a much smaller dose. Accprding to Rovesti and Gattefossé (1973) clary sage oil is mildly hypotensive. As the Shipchliev study employed the dosage level normally used in aromatherapy we may assume that clary sage is hypotensive. However, the possible influence of clary on adrenal secretion is very interesting, and may relate to its intoxicating effect.

An an anticonvulsive-euphoric-sedative clary is indicated in nervous, hysterical, paranoid, panicky states of mind and it is one of the very best remedies for depression, of whatever origin. It is a good tonic of the womb, and of the female function in general. (Perhaps, like garden sage, it contains oestrogens, or some similar substance.) In Joseph Miller's words clary 'helps to invigorate a cold, relaxed womb'. It is good for painful periods, for lack of, or scanty, menstruation, and is a useful oil for inhalation, fumigation, or compresses during childbirth. It encourages labour, at the same time helping the mother to relax.

Clary sage is renowned as a strengthener of the kidneys and stomach. Externally it cools inflammation, and is much used in skin care because of its scent. It is useful for inflamed, normal, or over-hydrated skin.

Cypress

Latin name	Cupressus sempervirens
Family	Coniferae
Quality	Yin
Ruling planet	Saturn
Evaporation rate	30
Odour intensity	4
Essence from	Fruit

Properties
Antiseptic
Antispasmodic
Antisudorific
Astringent
Deodorant
Diuretic
Hepatic
Sedative
Vasoconstrictor
  (local)

Uses
Asthma
Cancer?
Diarrhoea
Dysentery
Dysmenorrhoea
Enuresis
Haemorrhages
Haemorrhoids
Influenza
Liver disorders
Menopausal
  problems
Menorrhagia
Nervous tension
Pyorrhoea
Rheumatism
Skin care
Spasmodic cough
Varicose veins
Whooping cough

The cypress is a tall, conical-shaped tree. Its small flowers are succeeded by round cones, or nuts as they are called, which are coloured brown or greyish. Cypress trees are perennial, and originated in the East. They are commonly found in gardens and cemeteries of the Mediterranean region, and are also popular in English gardens and parks. The cypress gives its name to an island where it used to be worshipped.

Cypress oil is clear, and has a woody, nutty quality with a hint of spice — one of my favourite scents. It is more of a masculine fragrance, although some women may welcome it as a refreshing change from the heavy sweetness of most perfumes, and many other essences. Its scent is reminiscent of other oils

215

from the coniferous family — juniper and pine — and it blends well with them. It makes a relaxing and refreshing bath oil.

Culpeper has this to say of cypress:

> 'The cones, or nuts, are mostly used, the leaves but seldom; they are accounted very drying and binding, good to stop fluxes of all kinds, as spitting of blood, diarrhoea, dysentary, the immoderate flux of the menses, involuntery miction; they prevent bleeding of the gums, and fasten loose teeth: outwardly, they are used in styptic restringent fomentations and cataplasms.'

The Chinese do not distinguish clearly between *Thuja* and *Cupressus*. The following comments of Li Shih-Chên therefore refer to both species:

> 'The nuts are considered to be very nutritious and fattening, and they are said to benefit the respiratory organs and to check profuse perspiration. They also act on the liver, and are prescribed in convulsive disorders of children.'

Cypress oil is of benefit in conditions where there is excessive discharge of fluid, such as those mentioned by Culpeper. Its astringent and styptic quality also renders it useful in haemorrhages, such as haemoptysis and metrorrhagia; and externally for haemorrhoids, varicose veins, and oily skin. It appears to act on the female reproductive system, probably via the ovaries, and has proved to be of value in menopausal and menstrual disorders.

It is a powerful antispasmodic, and is very useful for asthma, whooping cough, and all spasmodic coughs. It is also a sedative of the nerve endings of the respiratory system (Couvreur). Due to this combined effect on the respiration cypress may also be of use in bronchitis and emphysema; its usefulness in influenza is already recognised (Valnet).

The action of cypress on the liver is not clear. It is unlikely to be of use in yin conditions, such as anaemia, but could be useful where there is excess heat or energy in the liver causing, for instance, an excess of bile. Because of its restringent effect on body fluids one would expect it to be most useful for the phlegmatic, loquacious type, for those with mental diarrhoea. Its effect on the nerves is sedative rather than stimulating.

Cypress would seem to be one of the most useful oils, if only we knew more about its properties. Its restraining effect on fluids is almost unique among essences. Its affinity for the female reproductive system (which may be due to a quasi-hormone) confirms its predominantly yin nature.

Eucalyptus

Latin name	*Eucalyptus globulus* and other species
Family	*Myrtaceae*
Quality	Yin
Ruling planet	Saturn
Evaporation rate	5
Odour intensity	8
Essence from	Leaves

Properties
Analgesic
Antiseptic
Antispasmodic
Cicatrisant
Deodorant
Depurative
Diuretic
Expectorant
Febrifuge
Hypoglycemiant
Rubefacient
Stimulant
Vermifuge
Vulnerary

Uses
Asthma
Bronchitis
Burns
Cancer?
Catarrh
Cholera
Colds
Cough
Cystitis
Diabetes
Diarrhoea
Diphtheria
Dyspepsia (atonic)
Emphysema
Fevers
Gall stones
Gonorrhoea
Haemorrhage

Herpes
Influenza
Leucorrhoea
Malaria
Measles
Migraines
Nephritis (acute)
Neuralgia
Pediculosis
Rheumatism
Scarlet fever
Sinusitis
Throat infections
Tuberculosos
Typhoid fever
Ulcers (skin)
Wounds

The eucalyptus tree (actually there are over 300 species) is one of the tallest trees in the world. *Eucalpytus amygdalin* sometimes grows up to 480 feet, even taller than the California Big Tree (*Sequoia gigantea*), and is probably the tallest tree in the world. *Eucalyptus globulus*, which is the best-known variety, attains heights of up to 357 feet. Like most of the eucalyptus family it is indigenous to the Australian continent.

The name comes from the Greek *eucalyptos*, meaning well-covered, because the flower buds are covered with a cup-like membrane which is thrown off as the flower expands. The leaves are tough and are shaped like a sword blade; they grow from six to twelve inches in length, being between one and two inches broad in the centre. They are a bluish-green colour, and usually have their edges vertically orientated. This would minimise the evaporation of essential oil and of water in the hot Australian sun.

It was Baron Ferdinand von Muller, a German botanist and explorer, who introduced the eucalyptus tree, along with its valuable essence, to the rest of the world. (From 1857 to 1873 he was director of the botanical gardens in Melbourne.) Since then it has been cultivated in many sub-tropical areas, including Egypt, Algeria, Spain, South Africa, India, and California. *Eucalyptus globulus* is still probably the most common variety, although there are now about fifty species cultivated for essential oil production. Those rich in eucalyptol (between 55% and 85%) are used in medicine and other species, which are chemically quite different, are used in perfumery.

The eucalyptus, or blue gum tree, has long been a favourite home remedy in Australia, the white settlers learning of its properties from the Aborigines. The following passage comes from Bill Wannan's *Folk Medicine*:

'In the latter half of the nineteenth century eucalyptus oil was regarded throughout the country as a general cure-all. May Gilmore wrote: "For every kind of wound made, father used eucalyptus leaves as taught by the blacks. Leaves were bound over blisters, burns, or scalds, and when in 1880 one of my brothers had his thumb nearly severed by an axe-cut, leaves bound on made such a good job of the healing that, though father had had to put in seven stitches, when a surgeon at last saw the hand he asked who had been the doctor, as he said no doctor could have done better." '

The eucalyptus plant was also widely used for colds, fevers, rheumatism, snake bites, dysentery, hay fever, neuralgia, and muscular aches and pains.

William Whitla comments

'Externally it is a rubefacient, and if covered with oiled silk it will blister. It is given in feverish septic conditions, and good results have followed its use in puerperal fevers, pyaemia, and septicaemia in five minim doses. It reduces the temperature, and has proved curative in ague, and during its elimination by the bronchial mucous surface and the renal tract it is a disinfecting expectorant in phthisis and bronchitis, and in cystitis and gonorrhoea. It has been given hypodermically in liquid vaseline.

'Many physicians are now treating all the exanthemata, pertussis, and diphtheria by enveloping the patient in an atmosphere of eucalyptus vapour. In influenza this has become the popular practice. Gurgenven has recently reported most favourably of the surprising results of this method of treating scarlatina.

'Locally the vapour has been used as an inhalation in gangrene of the lung, phthisis, ozaena, diphtheria, and a dilute solution is employed to wash out cavities and irrigate foul wounds. Made into a pessary, it has been used in cancer of the uterus and rectum, and as a gauze it is used as an antiseptic surgical dressing.'

'Eucalyptus oil is used as a stimulant and antiseptic gargle. Locally applied, it impairs sensibility. It increases cardiac action. Its antiseptic properties confer some anti-malarial action, though it cannot take the place of Cinchona.

'In croup and spasmodic throat troubles, the oil may be freely applied externally.

'In veterinary practice, Eucalyptus oil is adminis-tered to horses in influenza, to dogs in distemper, to all animals in septicaemia. It is also used for parasitic skin affections' (Mrs Grieve).

Eucalyptus oil is clear, is not much used in perfumery, but has a good reputation as an inhalant or chest rub. It has a distinctive camphoraceous odour, and a surprisingly bland, very slightly bitter taste. On the tongue is feels cold, like peppermint oil, although it contains no menthol.

The most salient quality of eucalyptus oil is its excellent action in all types of fever. The Aborigines use it as a febrifuge, Whitla recommends it for puerperal fevers, ague (intermittent fevers), exanthemata (eruptive fevers), and certain febrile conditions, such as diphtheria, influenza, and scarlet fever. Dr Valnet indicates its use in cholera, malaria, typhus, scarlatina, measles, and influenza. Eucalyptus has a pronounced cooling effect on the body, bringing about an effective reduction of temperature.

Eucalyptus is one of the best antiseptic oils, and its usefulness in many of the above conditions is also related to this quality. Its antiseptic efficacy is partly due to the formation of ozone which takes place on oxidation of some of its terpenes. The spraying of an emulsion containing 2% of eucalyptus oil kills off 70% of local, airborne staphylococci. According to Mrs Grieve it is an antimalarial antiseptic. An American study, published in 1958, showed eucalyptus to be moderately effective against *s.* typhosa, *p.* morgani, *b.* brevis, and *m.* citreus. A Russian study (1973) reveals that some eucalyptus oils (*e. viminalis, e. cinerea, e. macarthuri,* and *e. dalrympheana*) are effective against influenza viruses A_2 and A. Solutions up to 2% were tested on mice and ten-day-old chicken embryos.

Some species of eucalyptus yield a red gum, which exudes from the bark, and is known as *kino.* Eucalyptus oil possesses many of the qualities which are to be found in the oils extracted from gums, notably a pronounced effect in catarrhal or purulent discharges, genito-urinary and respiratory tract infections, and skin conditions. It is a very good remedy for indolent wounds and ulcers, and should be taken as a blood purifier in all conditions where there is any toxaemia or sepsis. Externally it is good for herpes and similar skin eruptions. It is a good analgesic in neuralgia, and an analgesic-cicatrisant for burns. As a rubefacient it may be applied externally for muscular or rheumatic pain, and is also a systemic remedy for rheumatoid arthritis. It may have a mild astringent effect.

Eucalyptus is best known for its action on the respiratory tract which is antiseptic, expectorant, and lightly antispasmodic.

221

It has proved a valuable remedy in most respiratory disorders, including sinusitis and tuberculosis, and is very good for most throat infections, especially when there is a heavy, mucousy discharge.

It also has a pronounced action on the urinary tract as an antiseptic and diuretic; it produces an increase in the excretion of urea. It is especially indicated where there is a putrescent, foul discharge and is valuable in cystitis, acute nephritis, leucorrhoea, and gonnorrhoea. It may also be used in acute diarrhoea and mucus.

Eucalyptus is especially indicated when there is sepsis, toxaemia, congestive headache, exhaustion, inability to concentrate, or fever. Because of its usefulness in colds, herpes, influenza, and measles eucalyptus would appear to be an acceptable anti-viral agent, *in vivo* if not *in vitro*. It has a slight oestrogenic effect, similar to fennel but less pronounced.

Fennel

Latin name	*Foeniculum vulgare*
Family	*Umbelliferae*
Quality	Yang
Ruling planet	Mercury
Evaporation rate	85
Odour intensity	6
Essence from	Seeds (they are actually fruits)

Properties
Antiseptic
Antispasmodic
Carminative
Diuretic
Emmenagogue
Expectorant
Galactagogue
Laxative
Splenetic
Stomachic
Tonic
Vermifuge

Uses
Alcoholism
Amenorrhoea
Colic
Constipation
Dyspepsia
Flatulence
Gout
Hiccough
Insufficient milk (of
    nursing mothers)
Kidney stones
Menopausal
    problems
Nausea
Obesity
Oliguria
Pulmonary ·
    affections
Vomiting

The name of fennel comes from the Latin *foenum*, meaning hay, and the Romans called it *foeniculum*. It grows four to five feet high, and has golden-yellow flowers. It is commonly found in Europe, and is thought to be indigenous to the shores of the Mediterranean. It flourishes particularly in limestone soil. Fennel was well known to the ancients, and was cultivated by the Romans. Pliny had great faith in its properties, and accorded at least twenty-two remedies to it. It is traditionally used in cooking, to combat obesity, and was said to convey strength, courage, and longevity. It is also said to strengthen the sight:

223

> 'Above the lower plants it towers,
> The fennel with its yellow flowers;
> And in an earlier age than ours
> Was gifted with the wondrous powers
> Lost vision to restore' (*Longfellow*).

In mediaeval times it was used to prevent witchcraft, and ward off evil spirits, and usually went by the name of *fenkle*.

> 'This herb is called fennel or fenkel. The virtue of this herb is thus. If the seed be dried, it is good, and comforteth the stomach. It openeth the stopping of the reins and of the bladder. If it be drunken with wine and water, it is good to do away with all manner venom. Also the juice dropped in the ears of a man, it will slay worms in a man. And also, if it be drunken with wine, it will break the dropsy and all manner swelling, and kepeth him from casting. And if it be drunken with wine and water, it maketh a woman's milk to increase. Also, if it be meddled with oil, it is good to heal a man's yard that is swollen. And this herb is hot and dry' (Banckes's *Herbal*).

> 'Fennel is good to break wind, to provoke urine, and ease the pains of the stone, and helps to break it. The leaves or seed, boiled in barley water, and drunk, are good for nurses to increase their milk, and make it more wholesome for the child . . . The seed, and the roots much more, help to open obstructions of the liver, spleen, and gall, and thereby ease the painful and windy swellings of the spleen, and the yellow jaundice; as also the gout and cramps. The seed is of good use in medicines, to help shortness of breath, and wheezing, by stopping of the lungs. It assists also to bring down the courses . . . Both leaves, seeds, and roots thereof are much used in drink or broth, to make people lean that are too fat' (Nicholas Culpeper).

> 'The seed is carminative, expelling wind, strengthening the bowels, and helping the colic, and is good to help a decayed sight' (Joseph Miller).

224

> 'The fruits are prescribed in fluxes, dyspepsia, colic, and other abdominal disorders of children. Made into a Spirit of Fennel, it is used locally for backache and toothache' (Li Shih-Chên).

Sweet fennel oil is one of the classic carminative remedies, and Joseph Miller mentions it as the only official preparation of fennel (1722). It is clear, has a sweet taste and an odour similar to aniseed. Like the other 'seed oils' fennel acts primarily on the digestive process. The oil does contain a small amount of ketones, but in normal doses presents no risk to epileptics.

Fennel is hot and dry to a moderate degree. It is good for weak, catarrhal constitutions, and is a tonic to the digestion, liver, and spleen. As an antispasmodic and expectorant it may be useful in bronchitis. It is an excellent remedy for all stomachic and digestive disorders, including flatulence, colic, all types of indigestion, nausea, and vomiting, and is reputed to be a hiccough remedy. On the evidence of several authorities fennel oil is both spasmodic and antispasmodic with regard to the intestine. The contractile effect, which accelerates and strengthens peristaltic movements, is beneficial in constipation, and helps whenever the colon is lacking in tone. The antispasmodic effect has resulted in its use in colic for hundreds of years. It is also used to prevent griping in combination with stronger purgatives. This apparent contradiction is due to a normalising, rather than a dose-dependent, effect. We can interpret it as a tonic quality, relieving abnormally strong spasm, and strengthening abnormally weak contractions. This would be a very good remedy for colitis and prolapsed colon.

Fennel is a good diuretic, and should be given when there is insufficient excretion of urine. It also helps to dissolve kidney stones. In spite of its ketone content it has a certain antitoxic effect. Culpeper mentions that fennel seed is 'good for those that are bit with serpents, or have eat poisonous herbs, or mushrooms', and Banckes's *Herbal* recommends it for 'all manner venom'. In recent times both tincture of fennel and anethole (the principal constituent of fennel oil) have been shown to reduce considerably the toxic effects of alcohol on the body.

In an experiment on mice, made to test the toxicity of fennel oil, relatively large doses were found to cause a reduction of body weight. The use of fennel for obesity is traditional, and would seem to indicate more than a diuretic effect; this may also be related to its hormonal action. It has been found to have an oestrogenic action, which is probably due to its anethole content. This indicates its use in menopausal problems, and is probably also related to the effect of fennel oil in increasing the milk of nursing mothers. In an experiment on goats it was found to increase both the quantity and the fat content of their milk. It will not, alas, help ladies who have no babies, but wish to increase their bust.

Frankincense

Latin name	*Boswellia thurifera*
Family	*Burseraceae*
Synonym	Olibanum
Quality	Yang
Ruling planet	Sun
Evaporation rate	75
Odour intensity	7
Essence from	Gum

Properties
Antiseptic
Astringent
Carminative
Cicatrisant
Digestive
Diuretic
Sedative
Tonic
Uterine
Vulnerary

Uses
Bronchitis
Carbuncles
Catarrh
Coughs
Dyspepsia
Gonorrhoea
Haemorrhage
Laryngitis
Leucorrhoea
Metrorrhagia
Scrofula
Skin care
Spermatorrhoea
Ulcers
Wounds

Gum frankincense, also known as olibanum (or occasionally 'gum thus'), and myrrh were the first gums to be used as incense. Frankincense was being imported by Egypt, from the land of Punt, nearly 5,000 years ago. It was used first as incense, and later in cosmetics and toiletries. In the form of incense it was also used to fumigate sick people, in order to drive out the evil spirits that were causing the sickness. The Egyptians did not use it for embalming purposes, but it was used in many of their rejuvenating face masks. Ovid, the Roman poet, in his book on skin care, *Medicamina Faciei*, includes frankincense as 'an excellent preparation for toilet purposes'.

Frankincense was one of the most highly prized substances of the ancient world. It has always been in plentiful supply, and has almost become synonymous with the term incense. In France it is known simply as *encens* (incense); the English word derives from the old French *franc encens*, frank here meaning luxuriant. In ancient times frankincense, in common with several other aromatics, was as valuable as gems or precious metals, hence the offering of gold, frankincense, and myrrh to the infant Christ. Its value was such that it had considerable influence on the economy of certain countries, and was often the cause of political dispute.

The gum comes from a small tree which grows in Arabia and Somaliland. It is extracted by making a deep incision in the trunk, below which a narrow strip of bark is peeled off. Over the following weeks a milky juice exudes, which slowly hardens on contact with the air. The tree has abundant leaves, and white or pale pink flowers.

Frankincense is mentioned in a French medical manuscript, written in the early thirteenth century:

> 'Olibanum ceo est encens, il est chaud et Seche el
> secunde de grei; il ad verru de conforter et de
> afermer, de traire ensemble, et de rettreindre. Il est
> bon, en auttre, les fermer des oyls et la dolur de
> denz, et encontre le hunel et encontre la grossesse
> et la rouillor des nariles et encontre in digestiun et
> amer eruc tuations et pur les mameles en greder un
> podre confit ad eysil e enplastre sur un dray e nus
> sur le mameles. roine chaude et seche el secunde de
> grei. Ele advertu a de faire e a degant. (Olibanum
> is known as frankincense, it is hot and dry in the
> second degree; it has the capacity to comfort and
> to fortify, to bring together, and to bind. It is also
> good for the shutting of the eyes, toothache, and
> against *le hunel* [?], pregnancy, soreness of the
> nostrils, and also indigestion and sour eructations.
> For the breasts, make up a powder prepared with
> vinegar and plaster on a sheet, and place it on the
> naked breasts. An excellent remedy, hot and dry in
> the second degree, it has the property of forming
> and [?]'.)

It is also mentioned in Banckes's *Herbal*:

'Olibanum is called frankincense. This is hot and dry in the third degree. It is a gum of a tree in India . . . It hath virtue of comforting by its sweet savour, also of closing and constraining. For the toothache that cometh of superfluity of humours from the head and especially by the veins, make a plaster of the powder of frankincense with wine and the white of an egg, meddle them together, and plaster them about the temples.

'Also, to stop the ways of the veins above, take frankincense and chew it well in thy mouth, and that shall stop and hinder the flux of humours coming down to the nostrils. Make pills of frankincense and swallow them down in the morning; then boil frankincense in wine, and at even drink that when thou goes to bed. Also these pills be good to help the digestion of the stomach, and good against sour belchings, also for the comforting and cleansing of the matrix, and helping of conception in the receiving the fume of frankincense beneath. Also, boil power of it in wine and when it is meetly [moderately] warm dip a cloth in it and lay it so warm to the share [pubes] of the patient, and greatly it comforteth the matrix.' [womb]

Joseph Miller comments:

'It is hot, dry, and binding, useful against diseases of the breast, as coughs, shortness of breath, catarrhous defluxions of rheum, and spitting of blood; it helps a looseness or a bloody flux, and stops a gonorrhoea and the whites; outwardly used in fumigations, it stops defluxions of rheum on the nostrils, and is good to cicatrise wounds and ulcers.'

Olibanum essence is reminiscent of camphor or turpentine, but also has a spicy, woody note, which gives it a much more pleasant smell than either of these. It is certainly a yang oil, and yet does not burn the tongue like benzoin, nor is it bitter like myrrh. It has a sweeter, lighter quality than either, and is more 'cephalic', more pleasing to the emotions. The oil is clear, and blends well with most other essences including camphor, sandalwood, pepper, and basil.

Not very much has been written about the medicinal virtues of frankincense since the eighteenth century. It seems to have fallen out of popularity, despite its comprehensive use by ancient civilisations. It is often said that it possesses the same properties as myrrh. The properties of the two certainly bear some similarity, but it is strange than an aromatic, especially one with such a reputation as frankincense, should have been so neglected. It may be inferior to myrrh in certain respects, as in treating mouth ulcers or inflammation, and this kind of comparison is probably the cause of its decline in therapy. It does, however, have some particular virtues of its own, not the least of these being its scent. For the reasons I have just outlined my sources of information here are pre-nineteenth century.

In common with most of the gum essences, frankincense has a pronounced effect on the mucous membranes, and is a very good expectorant. As an inhalation (and/or internally) it is a good remedy in all catarrhal conditions, whether of the head, lungs, stomach, or intestines. It has an affinity for the pulmonary and genito-urinary tracts, and is of use in coughs, bronchitis, laryngitis, shortness of breath; and also for leucorrhoea, gonorrhoea, and spermatorrhoea, and infections of the urinary tract such as cystitis and nephritis.

In China it has been used for scrofula (tuberculosis of the lymph glands) and for leprosy. Its astringent properties render it useful in haemorrhages, especially uterine or pulmonary. It is also good for the digestion, and for dyspepsia with sour belching. Externally it may be used for indolent wounds, ulcers, carbuncles, etc. in the same way as myrrh. It is good for all disorders of the uterus, and is safe to use in pregnancy and childbirth. Here is may be used internally, in douches, compresses, or fumigation. As an internal remedy, frankincense is much more pleasant to take than other gum essences.

In common with benzoin it has an elevating, warming, soothing effect on the mind and emotions. This recalls its traditional use in the driving away of evil spirits, if we think of these spirits rather as obsessions, fears, and anxieties which may have become manifest as physical illness.

Frankincense has also been widely used in skin care preparations in past centuries. It is astringent, may be slightly anti-inflammatory, and appears to preserve a youthful complexion, preventing (dare one say, slightly eradicating?) wrinkles and other abominations of old age.

Geranium

Latin name	*Pelargonium adorantissimum*
	Pelargonium graveolens
Family	*Geraniaceae*
Quality	Yin
Ruling planet	Venus
Evaporation rate	87
Odour intensity	6
Essence from	Herb

Properties
Analgesic
Antidepressant
Antiseptic
Astringent
Cicatrisant
Diuretic
Haemostatic
Sedative
Stimulant of
   adrenal cortex
Tonic
Vulnerary

Uses
Aphthae
Burns
Cancer (uterine)
Depression
Dermatitis
Diabetes
Diarrhoea
Eczema (dry)
Engorgement of
   breasts
Gastralgia
Glossitis
Haemorrhage
Jaundice
Kidney stones
Nervous tension
Neuralgia (facial)
Ophthalmia
Pediculosis
Ringworm
Shingles
Skin care
Sore throats
Sterility
Stomatitis
Ulcers (internal and
   external
Wounds

There are several aromatic pelargoniums. This variety grows about two feet in height, has serrated, pointed leaves, and small, pink, flowers. The whole plant is aromatic. It is found on waste land, in hedgerows, and on the outskirts of woods. It was used by the ancients as a remedy for wounds and tumours.

The essence is clear to light green, and has a delightfully

fresh scent. It makes a very refreshing and relaxing bath oil. It blends well with rose, citrus oils, and basil, but is one of the few oils that can be used in almost any blend. In small amounts it brings together the other scents, and gives a light, green, soft, and slightly floral quality to the whole. It has a bitter taste.

> 'It is under the dominion of Venus, and is commended against the stone, and to stay blood, where or however flowing; it speedily heels all green wounds, and is effectual in old ulcers in the privy parts, or elsewhere. All geraniums are vulneraries but this herb more particularly so, only rather more detersive and diuretic, which quality is discovered by its strong, soapy smell; it answers very well taken inwardly with wine in powder, and also outwardly applied, for old ruptures. A decoction of it has also been of service in obstructions of the kidneys and in gravel' (Nicholas Culpeper).

Geranium oil is predominantly yin but it also has a warming quality, not as a result of extreme yin becoming yang, but as a neutral oil inclining to the yin side. Its neutral quality is evidenced by its light green colour and explains why it blends so readily with almost any other oil.

It is a mild analgesic and sedative, and may be used for neuralgia, and when there is pain of perhaps more nervous than physical origin. As an analgesic-cicatrisant-antiseptic it is an excellent remedy for burns, and is renowned for its efficacy on wounds and all types of ulcers. Geranium reduces extremes of both yin and yang, and in wounds or other inflammatory conditions it will reduce inflammation. Where there is cold it has a mild stimulating effect. Its soothing action is of use in glossitis, ophthalmia, stomatitis, and gastro-enteritis.

The action of geranium on the nervous system is fairly pronounced. It is both sedative and uplifting, like bergamot, and is one of the essences successfully employed by Rovesti in the treatment of anxiety states. Like basil and rosemary, it is a stimulant of the adrenal cortex, whose hormones are essentially of a regulating, balancing nature. They also include sex hormones, and geranium may be used to balance hyposecretion of either androgens or oestrogens, such as often occurs during the menopause.

As an antiseptic, geranium is of average use, but is often effective in throat or mouth infections, where it also acts as an analgesic. It is binding and astringent, like cypress, and is very good for internal or external haemorrhages and diarrhoea. It may be useful for other fluxes such as blenorrhoea or leucorrhoea. Externally applied it is used for engorgement of the breasts.

It is an insecticide, due to its terpene content, and is very good as a mosquito repellent.

Geranium is a mild diuretic, and is used internally for stones of the urinary passages. It is also of value in jaundice, and its bitter taste indicates an effect on the small intestine. We can see this in its pronounced action on diarrhoea/enteritis; it may be effective against gall stones. It has also been used in the treatment of urinary tract disorders and tuberculosis.

It is a useful essence for all types of skin conditions including dry eczema, burns, shingles, ringworm, and pediculosis (lice). Geranium is also of great value in skin care, and can be used on almost any type of skin. It is cleansing, refreshing, astringent, and is a mild skin tonic. It may also be used on inflamed skin, and is good for sluggish, congested, oily types.

Hyssop

Latin name	*Hyssopus officinalis*
Family	*Labiatae*
Quality	Yang
Ruling planet	Jupiter
Evaporation rate	65
Odour intensity	6
Essence from	Herb

Properties
Antiseptic
Antispasmodic
Carminative
Cicatrisant
Digestive
Diuretic
Emmenagogue
Expectorant
Febrifuge
Nervine
Regulates blood
  pressure
Sedative
Sudorific
Tonic (especially
  heart and
  respiration)
Vermifuge
Vulnerary

Uses
Amenorrhoea
Asthma
Bronchitis
Bruises
Cancer?
Catarrh
Colic
Cough
Dermatitis
Dispnoea
Dyspepsia
Eczema
Fevers
Flatulence
Hypertension
Hypotension
Hysteria
Influenza

Leucorrhoea
Loss of appetite
Otitis
Quinsy
Rheumatism
Scrofula
Stones (urinary)
Syphilid
Tuberculosis
Whooping cough
Wounds

Hyssop is an unobtrusive little herb, usually found in dry, hilly places. It grows from one to two feet in height, and has slim,

234

pointed leaves, and pale blue flowers. It grows best in a warm, dry climate. It is one of the aromatic herbs mentioned in the Bible. Banckes's *Herbal* has this to say of the herb:

> 'Its virtue is, if a man takes the juice thereof, and put it in his mouth, it will heal all manner of evils in the mouth. Also, it slayeth worms in a mann's womb [belly] and maketh it soft. Also, if it be drunken green [fresh] or in powder, it maketh a man well-coloured. It is hot and dry.'

According to Culpeper:

> 'It is good to wash inflammations, and takes away the blue and black marks that come by strokes, bruises, or falls . . . It is an excellent medicine for the quinsy, or swelling in the throat, to wash and gargle it . . . The hot vapours of the decoction taken by a funnel in at the ears, eases the inflammations and singing noise of them . . . It is good for falling sickness [epilepsy], expectorates tough phlegm, and is effectual in all cold griefs, or diseases of the chest and lungs.'

Joseph Miller writes:

> 'Healing, opening, and attenuating, good to cleanse the lungs of tartarous humours, and helpful against coughs, asthmas, difficulty of breathing, and cold distempers of the lungs; it is likewise reckoned a cephalic, and good for diseases of the head and nerves.'

Essential oil of hyssop is a light golden-yellow colour, is fairly expensive, and is used in high-class perfumes and liqueurs; it is an important constituent of Chartreuse. The scent is difficult to describe because it is not like any other, and yet reminds one of many others, seeming to smell of a mixture of basil, geranium, and thyme. It is not as pleasant as geranium, but neither is it unpleasant. It has a hot, bitter taste, and a powerful effect on the mind, quickly clearing it of debris. It gives a feeling of alertness and clarity. It always reminds me of basil, and yet is not so quick or piercing.

Hyssop oil presents a certain toxicity due to its content of 'pino-camphone'. This is a ketone, and it is believed that high doses of ketones could bring on convulsions in people who are prone to epilepsy. However, if used in normal doses the oil is unlikely to present any risk. The old herbalists actually used to prescribe hyssop in the treatment of epilepsy, but of course they used the herb and not the oil. Knowing this, and given that the toxic effect of an oil is entirely relative to the amount used, we can assume that a small quantity, insufficient to produce a convulsive reaction, may be beneficial in cases of epilepsy and similar convulsive disorders.

Hyssop is a yang oil, and has a wide field of action which is basically stimulating. It has an unusual regulating effect on the blood pressure, tending to lower it if it is high, and raise it if it is low. In an experiment on dogs hyssop oil caused a small increase in blood pressure and respiration, followed by a decrease in blood pressure and an increase in heart rhythm, followed by a gradual return to normal. The effect is tonic, rather than stimulating. Jethro Kloss calls hyssop an 'excellent blood regulator and a fine tonic when the system is in a weakened condition'. He also recommends it for problems related to the spleen, and Mrs C. F. Leyel comments that hyssop 'is said to cure grief, through its action on the spleen'. Hyssop is an excellent tonic for disorders involving the cardiovascular system, and is of great value as a general tonic for convalescence.

Its action on the nervous system is similar in that it operates both as a mild sedative and as a nerve tonic. It strengthens and warms the nerves, bringing a feeling of relaxation. This strengthening or slightly stimulating effect can become convulsive in certain people. In hysteria, where there is no hint of epilepsy, it helps to depolarise yin and yang, bringing a state of relative normality.

Hyssop is very valuable in disorders of the respiratory tract; the essence is eliminated primarily via the lungs. It fluidifies mucus, promotes expectoration, and relieves bronchial spasm. It is an excellent cough remedy, and is also of great benefit in asthma, bronchitis, influenza and all catarrhal conditions. It is an effective anti-bacterial agent in tuberculosis, and is reputed to be of value in scrofula.

The effect of hyssop on the digestive system is perhaps of less interest. It is a mild laxative, relieves spasm, expels wind, promotes digestion, and kills worms. Externally applied it is very good for bruises and the like, for eczema, syphilis, and wounds. Hyssop oil is best avoided during pregnancy.

Jasmine

Latin name	Jasminum officinale
	Jasminum grandiflorum
Family	Jasminaceae
Quality	Yang
Ruling planet	Jupiter
Evaporation rate	95
Odour intensity	7
Essence from	Flowers

Properties
Antidepressant
Antiseptic
Antispasmodic
Aphrodisiac
Galactagogue
Parturient
Sedative
Tonic (especially
    uterine)

Uses
Anxiety
Cough
Depression
Dysmenorrhoea
Frigidity
Hoarseness
Impotence

Nervous chills
Skin care
Uterine disorders

Jasmine is one of the most expensive essences, and I have always felt that it deserves the title: 'King of Aromatics'. The name is derived from the Arabic *yasmin*. Chinese jasmine, *J. sambac*, is largely used for scenting tea; it is known in China as *mo li*, and the Hindus call it 'moonlight of the grove'. In China the flowers are used in cosmetics, to decorate the hair of pretty girls, and an infused oil was used in former times to massage the body after bathing.

The jasmine plant is a creeper, with white or yellow flowers. It is cultivated in Algeria, Morocco, France, China, Egypt, Italy and Turkey; the French oil is the most expensive. Jasmine oil

237

has for many years been extracted by enfleurage, although oils extracted by volatile solvents are now the only ones available. Jasmine is the most exquisite of scents, and is used in many of the costliest perfumes. The oil is a deep reddish-brown colour, a beautiful mahogany. It blends very well with rose, and with citrus oils. It has a sweet, exotic bouquet which never fails to please.

> 'Jessamine is a warm, cordial plant . . . It warms the womb, and heals Schirrthi therein, and facilitates the birth; it is useful for cough, difficulty of breathing, etc. It disperses crude humours, and is good for cold and catarrhous constitutions, but not for the hot.
>
> 'The oil is good also for hard and contracted limbs; it opens, warms and softens the nerves and tendons . . . It removes diseases of the uterus, and is of service in pituitous colics' (Nicholas Culpeper).

Jasmine oil works primarily on the emotional level, and is of great value in psychological and psychosomatic problems. Although it does have physiological effects, its use is espeically indicated when these are linked to an emotional problem. Jasmine is a nerve sedative, and at the same time greatly uplifting. It is anti-depressant, and produces a feeling of optimism, confidence, and euphoria. It is most useful in cases where there is apathy, indifference, or listlessness.

Like the rose, it has a marked effect on the female reproductive system. It relieves uterine spasm and also menstrual pain, whether in the abdomen or the back. It helps to relieve the pain of childbirth, and to promote the birth. It also promotes the flow of breast milk, and so is of great value as an ante- and post-natal massage oil. In Malaya seven jasmine flower are prescribed as a remedy for puerperal septicaemia. It is a notable aphrodisiac, warming and relaxing the body. Because of this, and because of its pronounced effect on the emotional sphere, jasmine is sometimes a great asset in treating impotence or frigidity. It also acts on the male sexual organs, warming and strengthening. It is useful in conditions where there is a discharge, such as spermatorrhoae, gonorrhoea, and prostatitis.

Jasmine oil acts on the respiration relieving cough, difficulty of breathing, hoarseness, nervous spasms at the back of the throat, and in the bronchi. It warms and strengthens a cold, weak stomach, and is of great value in general nervous debility, and conditions arising from it.

The action of jasmine is predominantly yang-warming, opening, relieving spasm. It is indicated where there is cold, listlessness, spasm, depression, catarrh or other discharge. It is, like all absolutes, a fairly powerful oil. There is no danger of toxicity but if it is over-used it will cease to be of benefit, and may result in an increase of catarrh. Too much yang eventually turns to yin.

Use in moderation, jasmine is beneficial for hot, dry, sensitive skins, especially if there is redness or itching. This does not preclude its use for other skin types, and because it is such a delicious scent it forms a welcome ingredient in any facial oil. It is sometimes of use in conditions such as dermatitis or erysipelas, especially when accompanied by depression.

Juniper

Latin name	*Juniperus communis*
Family	*Coniferae*
Quality	Yang
Ruling planet	Jupiter
Evaporation rate	30
Odour intensity	5
Essence from	Fruit (berries)

Properties

Antiseptic
Antispasmodic
Antitoxic
Aphrodisiac
Astringent
Carminative
Cicatrisant
Depurative
Diuretic
Emmenagogue
Nervine
Rubefacient
Sedative
Stomachic
Sudorific
Tonic
Vulnerary

Uses

Acne
Albuminuria
Amenorrhoea
Arteriosclerosis
Blenorrhoea
Cirrhosis
Colic
Cough
Cystitis
Dermatitis
Diabetes
Dropsy
Dysmenorrhoea
Dyspepsia (atonic)
Eczema
Flatulence
Gout

Haemorrhoids
Kidney stones
Leucorrhoea
Nervous disorders
Oliguria
Pulmonary
  infections
Pyelitis (chronic)
Rheumatism
Skin care
Strangury
Ulcers (external)
Urinary tract
  infections
Wounds

The juniper is a small evergreen tree or shrub with short, spiny leaves, closely arranged in whorls of three. It grows four to six feet in height, and is commonly found in chalky or limy soils. The oil is obtained from the berries which are small, like blackcurrants, and turn from green to a deep purple-blue when ripe. There is also an oil obtained from the wood, but it has much less therapeutic value.

Juniper was used to burn as incense by earlier civilisation. It was used in Tibet for both religious and medicinal purposes. Juniper was one of the many aromatic shrubs burned to ward off evil spirits, or to serve as a disinfectant in times of plague or other contagious diseases. The French used to burn a mixture of juniper twigs and rosemary leaves in hospital wards and sick rooms, to purify the air. In Yugoslavia juniper oil is almost a cure-all in their traditional folk-medicine.

The essence has a very slight greenish-yellow tinge, and a pleasant terebinthinate odour. Like oils of cypress and pine it makes a refreshing bath oil, and is both stimulating and relaxing. It has a fairly bitter taste. Juniper berries are used in making gin.

> 'The berries are hot in the third degree, and dry in the first, being counter-poison, and a resister of the pestilence, and excellent against the bites of venomous beasts; it provokes urine, and is available in dysenteries and strangury. It is a remedy against dropsy, and brings down the terms, helps the fits of the mother, expels the wind, and strengthens the stomach. Indeed there is no better remedy for wind in any part of the body, or the colic, than the chymical oil drawn from the berries. They are good for cough, shortness of breath, consumption, pains in the belly, rupture, cramps, convulsions . . . the berries stay all fluxes, help the haemorrhoids or piles, and kill worms in children' (Nicholas Culpeper).

By 'chymical oil' Culpeper means essential oil. It is mentioned in Joseph Miller's *Herbal* as the only official preparation of juniper.

> 'A mild stimulant and stomachic in small doses. It rapidly enters the blood, and is picked out by the kidneys, which it powerfully stimulates, carrying with it increased quantities of water if dropsy exist, while in health it may even diminish the quantity of water. It excites the genital organs and seems to resemble

cantharides when given in very large doses, as strangury and priapism have been known to follow its use' (William Whitla).

'The chief use of juniper is as an adjuvant to diuretics in dropsy, depending on heart, liver or kidney disease' (Mrs Grieve).

Juniper oil acts on the skin, digestion, urinary tract, the blood, and the nerves. Along with sandalwood it is one of the classic diuretics and remedies for urinary tract infections. It is also a good antiseptic for the respiratory tract, digestive tract, and blood. It is effective against meningococcus, staphylococcus, diphtheria bacillus, and Eberth's bacillus. It has been used in treatment for cholera, dysentery, and typhoid fever, although one cannot vouch for its antimicrobial properties in these cases.

A study on the diuretic action of juniper oil revealed that it acts by enhancing glomerular filtration, and that increased amounts of potassium, sodium, and chlorine are excreted. No adverse reactions were detected, and chronic administration of the oil produced no pathological changes.

The action of juniper resembles that of cypress, and they are quite closely related botanically. Cypress is definitely a more powerful astringent and antispasmodic, while juniper is a more effective diuretic. The diuretic and depurative actions of juniper make it an excellent remedy for rheumatism and gout. It may be used externally, suitably diluted in fatty oil, as a mild analgesic-rubefacient to relieve rheumatic pain. Its action on the urinary tract is of value in cystitis, chronic pyelitis, oliguria, and kidney stones. Like cypress, it is good for convulsive coughs, and has been used in Yugoslavian pharmacology for this purpose.

Juniper is an excellent remedy for colic and flatulence, and may be used for all types of indigestion, and minor stomach disorders. It has a strengthening, tonic effect on the nerves, and is indicated in nervous disorders, and states of stress and anxiety. Its sedative action will help those who find sleeping difficult because of worries and tensions. This, combined with its emmenagoguic action, makes it an appropriate remedy for lack of, or painful, menstruation. Culpeper recommends juniper for palsies (paralysis) and falling sickness (epilepsy);

Juniper stimulates the circulation, and as a blood purifier is indicated in all disorders of the skin and blood. It is equally useful applied externally for eczema, dermatitis, and perhaps psoriasis. Its combined depurative, sudorific, antiseptic, and rubefacient properties make it an ideal remedy for skin disorders. As an astringent it is good for haemorrhoids and all types of fluxes. As an antiseptic-astringent it is good for oily skins and acne. Juniper oil makes a very good aromatic water for cleansing and toning the skin.

Considering its relatively mild toxicity juniper is a remarkably effective and versatile remedy, with no contra-indications. It should be used in conditions characterised by cold, fear, trembling, weakness, and languor.

Lavender

Latin name	Lavandula angustifolia
	Lavandula officinalis
Family	Labiatae
Quality	Yang
Ruling planet	Mercury
Evaporation rate	85
Odour intensity	4
Essence from	Flowers

Properties
Analgesic
Anticonvulsive
Antidepressant
Antiseptic
Antispasmodic
Antitoxic
Carminative
Cholagogue
Choleretic
Cicatrisant
Cordial
Cytophylactic
Deodorant
Diuretic
Emmenagogue
Hypotensor
Nervine
Sedative
Splenetic
Sudorific

Uses
Abscess
Acne
Alopecia areata
Asthma
Blenorrhoea
Blepharitis
Boils
Bronchitis
Burns
Carbuncles
Catarrh
Chlorosis
Colic
Conjunctivitis
Convulsions
Cystitis
Depression
Dermatitis
Diarrhoea
Diphtheria

Dyspepsia
Earache
Eczema
Epilepsy
Fainting
Fistula (anal)
Flatulence
Gonorrhoea
Halitosis
Headache
Hypertension
Hysteria
Influenza
Insomnia
Laryngitis
Leucorrhoea
Migraine
Nausea
Nervous tension
Neurasthenia

Properties	Uses
Tonic	Oliguria
Vermifuge	Palpitations
Vulnerary	Paralysis
	Pediculosis
	Psoriasis
	Rheumatism
	Scabies
	Scrofula
	Stones (gall)
	Sunstroke
	Throat infections
	Tuberculosis
	Typhoid fever
	Ulvers (cornea, leg)
	Vomiting
	Whooping cough
	Wounds

The word lavender comes from the Latin *lavare*, meaning to wash. It was one of the favourite aromatics used by the Romans in connection with their bathing activities. They probably introduced the plant to England, and ever since then it has been a great favourite with women. It is widely used as a toilet water, and forms the principal ingredient of many pot-pourris and sachets. In earlier times it was used to strew the floors of houses and churches on festive occasions, and was very popular in toilet waters and vinegars.

Lavender is cultivated in many European countries, but the main producer is France. A good quality oil is also produced in Tasmania. English lavender oil, although well-known in name, is produced only on a very small scale, principally in Norfolk, and it has a distinctly camphoraceous odour. The original English lavender used to be cultivated in Mitcham, Surrey.

The fresh, clean scent of lavender needs no description, neither does the plant. The essence is widely used in perfumery, especially in toilet waters, and is still an extremely popular scent. The oil is clear, and has a fairly mild, bitter taste. It blends well with a great number of essences, adding a light, floral softness to almost any mixture.

'This is called lavender. If this be sodden in water, give that water to drink to a man that hath the palsy, and it will heal him. It is hot and dry' (Banckes's *Herbal*).

'The distilled water of lavender smelt unto, or the temples and forehead bathed therewith, is a refreshing to them that have the Catalepsy, a light migram, and to them that have the falling sicknesse, and that use to swoune much . . . It profiteth them much that have the palsie, if they be washed with the distilled water of the floures, or anointed with the oile made of the floures, and oile olive, in such a maner as oile of Roses is, which shall be expressed in the treatise of Roses' (John Gerarde).

'Lavender is almost wholly spent with us, for to perfume linnen, apparell, gloves and leather and the dryed flowers to comfort and dry up the moisture of a cold braine . . . This is usually put among other hot herbs, either into bathes, ointment or other things that are used for cold causes' (John Parkinson).

'Mercury owns this herb. It is of especial use in pains of the head and brain which proceed from cold, apoplexy, falling-sickness, the dropsy, or sluggish malady, cramps, convulsions, palsies, and often faintings. It strengthens the stomach, and frees the liver and spleen from obstructions, provokes women's courses, and expels the dead child and afterbirth. The flowers if steeped in wine help those to make water that are stopped, or troubled with the wind or colic, if the place be bathed therewith . . . Two spoonfulls of the distilled water of the flower help them that have lose their voice, the tremblings and passions of the heart, and fainting and swoonings, applied to the temples or nostrils, to be smelt unto' (Nicholas Culpeper).

Lavender is generally regarded as the most useful and versatile essence for therapeutic purposes. Its properties show a fairly equal balance between yin and yang, and in this context it is virtually neutral. It has a sedative and tonic action on the heart (hysteria, nervous tension, palpitations) and lowers high blood-pressure. It is a mild local analgesic, and calms cerebro-spinal excitability; it is renowned for its nervine-sedative properties, and has proved valuable in a variety of nervous and psychological disorders, including depression, insomnia, migraine, hysteria, nervous tension, and paralysis. As a sedative-analgesic it is very good for headache and migraine. Lavender is rather like geranium, in that it has a predominantly normalising, rather than yin or yang quality, hence its considerable versatility. It may be used in epilepsy, convulsions, catalepsy, and other nervous conditions caused by a serious imbalance of yin and yang. It is a heart tonic, and calms the nerves of the heart. Culpeper's 'tremblings and passions of the heart' very aptly describes the kind of mental state in which lavender is indicated: palpitation, trembling, irritability, fainting, panic, hysteria (first deciding one thing, then equally firmly deciding the opposite). Mrs Grieve mentions the use of lavender tincture for delusions and mental depression. Lavender should be used whenever there are strong mental symptoms, with a picture of constant change from one extreme to the other, such as in manic depression. It is very good for nervous exhaustion.

Although it is not really anti-inflammatory, lavender is often useful where there is inflammation, hence its use in burns, dermatitis, eczema, psoriasis, boils, rheumatism, wounds, ulcers, blepharitis, conjunctivitis, cystitis, diarrhoea, laryngitis, and so on. In most of these conditions its antiseptic properties are also of value. It is good for catarrhal discharges (leucorrhoea, gonorrhoea, bronchitis, etc.), and is also a mild analgesic, which enhances it value in most of the above conditions. It is good for rheumatic or muscular aches and pains, and is a useful ingredient for massage oils, especially for athletes and sportsmen.

Lavender is a good antispasmodic (asthma, bronchitis), carminative, and stomachic (colic, nausea, vomiting, flatulence, dyspepsia), especially when these conditions are associated with nervous or emotional problems. It increases gastric secretion and intestinal motility. Its antiseptic properties are especially suited to combating halitosis, and it is an excellent skin antiseptic.

It may be used in any skin condition (dermatitis, eczema, acne, psoriasis, etc.) and is also effective against certain skin parasites (lice, scabies). It has proved to be an effective remedy in some cases of alopecia areata, and may be used for all types of baldness, especially when associated with nervous problems. It may be used with benefit on any type of skin (oily, dry, sensitive, acneic) although it seems to work best in combination with other essences. It is a very good cytophylactic (regeneration of skin cells) and so may be considered as a skin-rejuvenating agent. This quality also explains why lavender is probably the most effective essence for burns. It is a pleasant and effective deodorant.

As an antiseptic-antiphlogistic-cicatrisant lavender is one of the best oils to use on inflamed, infected wounds and ulcers. Dr Valnet recommends its use for syphilitic chancres, gangrenous wounds, and anal fistulas. As an antiseptic lavender may be used for most throat infections, and is often useful in influenza. As an antiseptic-diuretic it is very good for cystitis, especially when associated with cold or colds. It is indicated when there is an abnormally low excretion of urine.

Lavender oil is an excellent remedy for sunstroke, and, made up as a massage oil, will help to prevent burning. However it is not an effective sun-screening agent, and is not sufficient when bathing in very strong sunlight.

Lavender is good for ulcerative lesions of the cornea. It produces arterial hypotension, and decreases the surface tension of the blood. It is a central nervous system depressant, and inhibits spontaneous motor activity. It inhibits mycobacterium tuberculosis, staphylococcus, gonococcus, Leoffler's bacillus (diphtheria), Eberth's bacillus (typhoid); lavender oil vapour destroys pneumococcus and haemolytic streptococcus within twelve to twenty-four hours. It has a very low toxicity.

It is a useful remedy for infants, especially in treating colic, nervous excitement, irritability, general debility, cutaneous affections, and infections in general. It is said to be good for whooping cough, but I do not know of any cases where it has been used on infants with this condition. Lavender is particularly useful for ear, nose, and throat infections, and is a useful alternative to camomile for infantile earache.

Lavender oil is useful in various procedures during childbirth. It makes for a speedy delivery without increasing the severity of contractions. It helps to calm the mother, and, as an aromatic water, may be used as a refreshing compress for the head. It may be used in an oil to massage the lower back (which also minimises pain) and in a warm compress over the abdomen. It also helps to expel the afterbirth. A few drops on a source of heat will refresh and purify the air. As an emmenagogue lavender is good for scanty menstruation, and may be useful for period pains. It is an excellent remedy for leucorrhoea, used in vaginal douches.

Used externally, it is one of the most effective oils for stimulating leucocytosis. Lavender should be considered whenever there is infection, spasm, inflammation, or emotional/nervous disturbance. Although several herbalists have referred to the toxicity of lavender oil, it is in fact one of the least toxic of all essences, and is less toxic even than camomile oil. The effects of lavender are usually enhanced by blending with other essences.

When using lavender for inflammatory conditions use only low concentrations (less than 1%). In higher concentrations it has more of a stimulating effect on the circulation. When being used for muscular aches, sprains and strains, rheumatic pains, etc. use between 2% and 4%. When using lavender on inflamed wounds, ulcers, skin conditions, or similar inflammations, it is usually best to blend it with camomile.

A lavender bath is refreshing, relaxing, and almost inevitably therapeutic, whatever the case. It warms the heart, and steadies the emotions, and makes a very good evening bath for those who have difficult in sleeping. In many ways lavender is similar to camomile but it is less toxic and more neutral, camomile being fairly yin. A warm lavender bath or footbath is very good for relieving physical or nervous fatigue.

Lavender oil is a very effective remedy for insect bites and stings, particularly those of the bee, wasp, gnat and mosquito, and it is equally effective against nettle stings. Rub a little neat lavender directly onto the sting or bite.

Marjoram

Latin name	*Origanum marjorana*
Family	*Labiatae*
Quality	Yang
Ruling planet	Mercury
Evaporation rate	40
Odour intensity	5
Essence from	Herb

Properties
Analgesic
Anaphrodisiac
Antiseptic
Antispasmodic
Carminative
Cordial
Digestive
Emmenagogue
Expectorant
Hypotensor
Laxative
Nervine
Sedative
Tonic
Vulnerary

Uses
Arthritis
Asthma
Colds
Colic
Constipation
Dysmenorrhoea
Dyspepsia
Flatulence
Genital erethism
Headache
Hypertension
Hysteria
Insomnia
Leucorrhoea
Migraine

Nervous tension
Neurasthenia
Tic

Marjoram is a familiar culinary herb, and also has a great reputation as a herbal medicine. It was widely used by the ancient Greeks, in medicines, perfumes, and other toiletries. They used it as a remedy for convulsions, dropsy, and narcotic poisoning. In England it used to be known as *magerum* or *margerome*. The origin of the word is uncertain, but perhaps derives from the Greek *margaron* meaning pearl, which has given us the name Margaret. The name origanum derives from the Greek *oros* (mountain) and *ganos* (joy).

Like basil, marjoram has a more refined scent than most of the essential oils from labiates. It blends well with lavender and bergamot, and the three oils together produce a very pleasant relaxing blend. Its taste is extremely bitter, and it warms the heart and stomach. Marjoram makes a relaxing, warming, and fortifying bath oil.

> 'This herb is hot and dry in the second degree . . .
> It hath vertue of comforting, of loosing, of consum-
> ing, and of cleansing. If the powder of it be drunken
> in wine — or else boil the powder of it in wine — it
> will heat well a stomach. Also, it comforteth the
> digestion. Also, take the leaves and flowers of
> magerum and pound them a little, and make the hot
> in a pan, and lay it to the grievance, and it taketh
> away the disease in the stomach that cometh of wind.
> Also, for the rheum in the head take this herb and
> bind it warm about thy head. Also, it dryeth the
> mother [womb] and consumeth the superfluity of it'
> (Banckes's *Herbal*).

> 'Our Common Sweet Marjoram is warming and
> comforting in cold diseases of the head, stomach,
> sinews [muscles] and other parts, taken inwardly or
> outwardly applied. The decoction thereof being
> drunk, helps diseases of the chest, obstructions of the
> liver and spleen, old[1] griefs of the womb, and the
> windiness thereof, and the loss of speech, by resolu-
> tion of the tongue . . . It provokes women's courses,
> if put up as a pessary . . . The oils is very warm and
> comforting to the joints that are stiff, and the sinews
> that are hard, to mollify and supple them' (Nicholas
> Culpeper).

> 'A cephalic plant, appropriated to the head and
> nerves . . . as convulsions, apoplexy, palsy, vertigo,
> headache and the like' (Joseph Miller).

Marjoram oil is predominantly yang, and sedative. It warms, relieves spasm, aids digestion and menstruation, and lowers

1 Almost certainly a misprint for 'cold'.

high blood pressure; it stimulates the parasympathetic nervous function and lowers the sympathetic function, resulting in general vasodilation. Most of its functions centre around this action on the autonomic nervous system. Its antispasmodic-sedative-warming effect makes it a very useful ingredient for body massage oils for general application. Culpeper even recommends it for 'places out of joint'.

Culpeper sees this warming effect as being useful for diseases of almost any part of the body which are related to coldness or spasm. Many essences can be described as warming, but there is something special about the comforting effect of marjoram. Notice how Culpeper refers to cold 'griefs' of the womb. Marjoram is very good for conditions coming from grief, and has an especially warming, comforting effect on the heart; by causing vasodilation it relieves the burden or pressure on the heart allowing it to rest. Its extremely bitter taste hints at an affinity with the heart. John Gerarde suggests marjoram 'for those who are given to over-much sighing'.

Externally applied marjoram is warming and analgesic, and is good for muscle spasm, rheumatic pains, sprains, strains, and so on. It also helps to disperse bruises. For colds it may be used in inhalations, or massaged over the sinus areas and temples. For headaches and migraines it may also be taken internally. As a warming emmenagogue it should be used in vaginal douches, and is good for leucorrhoea and painful periods.

Marjoram is a very good remedy for excessive sexual impulses. This in itself may not be seen as an abnormality or a disease, but the property has been held to be part of the character of the herb since its discovery by a clergyman who had an asylum for orphans. It may be useful in nocturnal orgasm, obsessive masturbation, nymphomania, etc., especially when associated with hysteria or anxiety.

Marjoram acts as a laxative by stimulating and strengthening intestinal peristalsis; this also relates to its digestive and carminative action. At the same time it relieves intestinal spasm, and so is useful for colic, flatulence, and spasmodic indigestion. Its action on the nervous system is sedative and tonic. It is effective for insomnia and states of anxiety, especially when there is high blood pressure, and has been successfully used for tics and hysteria. Marjoram oil is best avoided during pregnancy.

Melissa

Latin name	*Melissa officinalis*
Family	*Labiatae*
Synonyms	Balm, lemon balm
Quality	Yang
Ruling planet	Jupiter
Evaporation rate	?
Odour intensity	4?
Essence from	Herb

Properties
Antidepressant
Antispasmodic
Carminative
Cordial
Digestive
Febrifuge
Hypotensive
Nervine
Sedative
Stomachic
Sudorific
Tonic
Uterine
Vermifuge

Uses
Allergies
Asthma
Colds
Colic
Depression
Dysentery
Fevers
Indigestion
Hypertension
Menstrual
    problems
Migraine
Palpitations
Nausea

Nervous tension
Shock
Sterility (in women)
Vertigo
Vomiting

Melissa leaves have a delightful, lemony scent, and the plant is often referred to as 'lemon balm'. Compared with lemon oil, melissa has a more delicate, herbal scent which is quite unique. Melissa is found in Europe, Middle Asia and North America. It is common in England and rapidly spreads whether cultivated or wild. The leaves are small and serrated, and the flowers are

253

white or yellow. The scent is most powerful in early summer, just before the blossom appears.

The name melissa is from the Greek word for 'bee', an insect which finds melissa flowers particularly good for making honey, and is attracted by the scent of the plant. The name 'balm' is an abbreviationo of balsam, and shows that it has been known for its scent since it was first named. It is one of our earliest medicinal herbs, and was highly esteemed by Paracelsus, who called it the elixir of life, and combined it with carbonate of potash in a mixture known as *primum ens melissae*. The essence has been in medicinal use since the late seventeenth century.

All the old herbalists extolled its virtues as a remedy for melancholy and a strengthener of the brain and nerves. Joseph Miller wrote:

> 'It is good for all disorders of the head and nerves;
> cheers the heart, and cures the palpitation thereof;
> prevents fainting, melancholy, hypochondriac and
> hysteric disorders, resists putrefaction, and is of use in
> malignant and contagious distempers.'

He also recommends it for bee and wasp stings. John Gerarde has this to say:

> 'The later age, together with the Arabians and
> Mauritanians, affirme Balme to be singular good for
> the heart, and to be a a remedy against the infirmities
> thereof; for Avicen in his booke written of the infir-
> mities of the heart, teacheth that Bawme makes the
> heart merry and joyful and strengtheneth the vitall
> spirits.'

Culpeper is even more informative:

> 'It is an herb of Jupiter, and under Cancer, and
> strengthens nature much in all its actions . . .
> Seraphio saith, it causeth the mind and heart to
> become merry, and reviveth the heart, faintings and
> swoonings, especially of such who are overtaken in
> sleep, and driveth away all, troublesome cares and
> thoughts out of the mind, arising from melancholy

and black choler: which Avicen also confirmeth.

'It is very good to help digestion, and open obstructions of the brain . . . it is good for the liver and spleen.'

It is noteworthy that both these authors associate the physical heart with the emotional heart.

The action of this oil is tonic, rather than stimulant; it is a tonic to the heart, nervous and digestive systems, and the uterus. It is sedative, calming, antidepressant. It slows the respiration and pulse, lowers the blood pressure, and has an antispasmodic effect on smooth muscle.

Its effect on the heart is tonic and antispasmodic, and the opposite to a cardiac stimulant. It slows the heart and relieves spasm; hence its usefulness in palpitation. It would appear that melissa may be of some use in all heart conditions where there is overstimulation, or heat, leading to weakness of the heart, and so to pathological change.

Closely related to its cardiac action is the effect of melissa oil on the nervous system. It is through the nervous system that it manifests a hypotensive and antispasmodic action. It is powerfully sedative, and at the same time, partly through its release of tension and spasm, has that uplifting, joyful effect on the spirit so common to aromatic oils. Its use in nervous disorders is especially related to over-sensitivity, leading to a constant, panicky type of anxiety. It is indicated in all hysterical or nervous affections.

As a digestive-stomachic-carminative the action of melissa oil closely resembles that of peppermint or fennel. Again its principal characteristic is tonic rather than stimulant; by relieving spasm it allows a natural flow of digestive juices. It is excellent for nausea, vomiting, and indigestion, especially of a nervous origin, and is undoubtedly of use in flatulence.

In cases of fever it induces a mild perspiration and has a cooling effect. For this reason it is of value in colds and influenza. Also of benefit here is its antispasmodic effect on the bronchi, which renders it useful for asthma and possibly bronchitis. It has a yin effect on the respiration, slowing it down, relieving spasm, and cooling excess heat.

Melissa seems to have an affinity for the female reproductive system. It as a mild emmenagoguic action, and is useful for painful periods. In both these cases one can see the soothing, relaxing, antispasmodic effect at work. Through helping, or permitting, nature to function in her own rhythm by removing tensions and blocks, melissa is also of great use in menstrual irregularity and female infertility.

The overall effect of melissa is that of a gentle but effective general tonic, a mild yang remedy. Because of its notable effect on the heart, blood pressure, nervous system, and, intimately related to these, the emotions, melissa is the nearest one can find to a rejuvenator — not something which will make us young again, but which helps to cushion the effect of our mind and the world outside, on our body. Perhaps Paracelsus was not so wrong when he called it the elixir of life!

Myrrh

Latin name	Commiphora myrrha
	Balsamodendron myrrha
Family	Burseraceae
Quality	Yang
Ruling planet	Sun
Evaporation rate	100?
Odour intensity	7
Essence from	Gum

Properties
Antiseptic
Antiphlogistic
Astringent
Carminative
Emmenagogue
Expectorant
Sedative
Stimulant (especially pulmonary)
Stomachic
Tonic
Uterine
Vulnerary

Uses
Amenorrhoea
Aphthae
Catarrh
Chlorosis
Cough
Diarrhoea
Dyspepsia
Flatulence
Gingivitis
Haemorrhoids
Leucorrhoea
Loss of appetite
Pyorrhoea
Stomatitis
Thrush
Tuberculosis
Ulcers (mouth, skin)
Wounds

Gum myrrh (from which the oil is extracted) exudes from the branches of the myrrh bush, either when it is wounded or from natural fissures. It flows out as a thick pale yellow liquid, and turns reddish-brown as it dries and hardens. The myrrh bush does not grow more than nine feet tall; it has sturdy, knotted branches, trifoliate leaves (which are also aromatic), and small, white flowers. It grows in north-east Africa, in very dry conditions, and is most commonly found in southern Arabia. It is

257

also to be found in the 'Garden of Eden' — the land between the rivers Tigris and Euphrates, which was part of Babylonia in the time of Moses. This is not generally reckoned to be the myrrh of the Bible, although there is so much uncertainty about the matter that it could in fact be so.

Myrrh was probably more widely used in ancient times than any other aromatic for incense, perfumes, and medicines. Its popularity as a perfume is not easy to understand, as it is not the sweetest of oils. It has a musty, balsamic, incense-like smell, and gives a pleasant smoky background to blends when used in small quantities. The essence is a beautiful reddish-brown colour.

At Heliopolis the ancient Egyptians used to burn myrrh at noon every day as part of their sun-worshipping ritual. They also used it extensively in the embalming of corpses, primarily to fill the stomach. Because of its ability to preserve the flesh myrrh oil is of some use as a cosmetic ingredient. It will not make wrinkles miraculously disappear, but is said to help preserve a youthful complexion. Egyptian women undoubtedly used it themselves in facial masks and other concoctions. It has a slightly cooling effect on the skin, and so would be especially useful in such a hot, dry climate. The Book of Esther relates that six of the twelve months devoted to the purification of women were accomplished with oil of myrrh.

One of the most celebrated perfumes of ancient Greece was known as *megaleion*, and included myrrh oil in its composition. It was also used for its healing properties, especially for applying to battle-wounds to promote healing and reduce inflammation. According to Greek legend myrrh was believed to have originated from the tears of 'Myrrha', daughter of Cinyrus, King of Cyprus, who had been metamorphosed into a shrub.

Joseph Miller, is very informative regarding the properties of myrrh:

> 'Myrrh is of an opening, heating, drying nature, resists putrefaction, and is of great service in uterine disorders, openng the obstruction of the womb, procuring the menses, expediting the birth, and expelling the secundines. It is good likewise for old coughs and hoarseness, and the loss of voice, and is very useful against pestiltial and infectious distempers, both taken inwardly, and flung upon burning coals and the fume received.

'Outwardly applied it cures wounds and ulcers, and prevents gangreens and mortifications.'

Li Shih-Chên says:

'It is regarded as an alterative and sedative, and, as formerly in the West, is used in the treatment of wounds and ulcers. It is thought to be especially useful in uterine discharges and in vicious lochiae; also in the treatment of a disease resembling hysterical mania.'

Richard Lucas in *Nature's Medicines* cites rubbing the body with tincture of myrrh as a means of protection against cold, saying that it:

'strengthens and improves the condition of the skin. This practice is useful especially in cases where the skin is relaxed and the patient feeble, as in chronic bronchitis, chronic pleurisy, asthma, chronic rheumatism, chronic diarrhoea, marasmus, and in every other form of disease attended by general debility.'

Myrrh oil is not very heating — indeed it is anti-inflammatory — but it is basically yang in nature. It is stimulating and strengthening, and its main area of action is the pulmonary system. It is particularly indicated in yin states where there is wasting or degeneration, such as indolent wounds and ulcers, gangrene, pyorrhoea, tuberculosis, and phthisis pulmonalis (a wasting disease of the lungs). It is almost as if this deep red essence has captured the life-giving strength of the North African sun.

Myrrh oil is a very good expectorant and as such it is of value in coughs, bronchitis, colds, and any condition involving an excess of thick mucus, not only promoting the evacuation of mucus but soothing the inflamed mucous membranes. Myrrh is not only of use in bronchial mucous conditions, but also in leucorrhoea, diarrhoea, and other related discharges.

Its action on the digestive system is stimulant and carminative, exciting the appetite and the flow of gastric juice and correcting flatulence. It is useful for weak stomachs where the food is prone to ferment. By correcting this state myrrh helps to eliminate foul breath, which is usually due to poor digestion and unnatural fermentation. The action of myrrh on the throat and mouth is quite pronounced: it is an excellent remedy for mouth ulcers, inflammation of the mouth (stomatitis), and pyorrhoea. Jethro Kloss also recomends it for diphtheria, Wren for thrush, and Joseph Miller for loss of voice.

The efficacy of myrrh for indolent wounds and ulcers is legendary. This is probably due to a combination of antiseptic, astringent, and antiphlogistic properties. Its astringency also renders it useful as an external application for haemorrhoids. It is recommended by Mrs Grieve for chlorosis, a type of anaemia accompanied by a greenish complexion, to which young women are particularly susceptible.

The myrrh bush must be very hardy to be able to survive in the desert. Myrrh oil is equally strong, equally powerful; at the same time it is very safe to use, and perhaps more than any other aromatic has stood the test of time. It has been used by many people, in many ways, for at least 3,000 years, and is still a very popular remedy. Myrrh oil is best avoided during pregnancy.

Orange Blossom (Neroli)

Latin name	*Citrus aurantium*
Family	*Rutaceae*
Quality	Yang
Ruling planet	Sun
Evaporation rate	79
Odour intensity	5
Essence from	Flowers

Properties	**Uses**
Antidepressant	Depression
Aphrodisiac	Diarrhoea (chronic)
Antiseptic	Hysteria
Antispasmodic	Insomnia
Cordial	Nervous tension
Deodorant	Palpitations
Digestive	Shock
Sedative	Skin care
Tonic	

There are two types of orange tree, the sweet orange, *Citrus sinensis*, and the bitter orange, *Citrus aurantium*. Oil of orange blossom, which is known as neroli oil, is extracted from the white blossoms of the bitter orange. Sweet orange flowers also yield an essence but it is of an inferior quality, and is not much used. The origin of the name neroli is uncertain. It is thought by some to originate from the name of the Emperor Nero, but the most generally accepted theory is that it stems from a certain Anne-Marie, Princess of Nerola, who first used it to perfume her gloves and her bath water. She was the wife of a famous Italian prince who lived in the sixteenth century; her glove perfume became very popular and gloves scented with it were known as *guanti di Neroli*.

It is thought that orange trees first reached Europe in the twelfth century, brought by Portuguese sailors from the East

Indies. The orange tree is a native of China, where the flowers have been used for centuries in cosmetic preparations. It is now cultivated in France, Tunisia, Italy, and the USA. The two types of orange tree strongly resemble each other, except that the leaf stalk of the bitter orange bears a small 'second leaf' which, when flattened out, forms a perfectly shaped heart.

Neroli oil is, as its price suggests, among the finest of flower essences. Its most common use is in Eau-de-Cologne, where it blends with lavender, bergamot, lemon, and rosemary to form the classic toilet water. It will also blend with sandalwood, jasmine, and rose, and is good to use as the 'heart' of a floral blend. It has an exquisite, sweet, feminine odour which is as unique as rose or jasmine, and not easy to describe; perhaps it most closely resembles lavender oil. It is a pale yellow colour, and has a bitter taste, indicating a possible action on the heart and small intestine.

Neroli is one of the most effective sedative-antidepressant oils: it may be used for insomnia, hysteria, states of anxiety and depression. It calms and slows down the mind. It also has a notable action on the heart, diminishing the amplitude of heart muscle contraction, hence its use in palpitations or other types of cardiac spasm. Derived from this is its use in panicky, hysterical, fearful types of people — those who upset themselves unnecessarily, and become overwrought over nothing. One can also see that neroli is a valuable remedy for shock, or for disorders caused by sudden shock, or fear, causing a strain on the heart. It is valuable in chronic diarrhoea, when this is related to long-standing stress or fear. Its action is slow but sure.

Oil of neroli also has a pronounced action on the skin. Like lavender and geranium it can be used with benefit on any type of skin. It is totally non-irritant and may be used where there is irritation or redness. It is said to be useful for dry broken skin and broken veins. It is one of the oils which acts on a cellular level, stimulating the elimination of old cells and the growth of new ones. Neroli makes a luxurious, relaxing, and deodorant bath oil.

Orange-flower water is soothing, digestive, carminative. It makes a very useful, mild remedy for infants' colic, and its sedative action helps to send them to sleep.[1]

1 See page 309.

Patchouli

Latin name	*Pogostemon patchouli*
Family	*Labiatae*
Quality	Yang
Ruling planet	Sun
Evaporation rate	100
Odour intensity	5
Essence from	Herb

Properties
Antidepressant
Antiphlogistic?
Antiseptic
Aphrodisiac
Astringent?
Cicatrisant
Deodorant
Sedative
Tonic

Uses
Anxiety
Depression
Skin care
Wounds

Patchouli comes from India, where it is known as *puchaput*. The plant is of the labiate family, but the oil is unlike other labiate oils. The leaves of patchouli are ovate, about four inches long and five inches broad. The stems grow up to three feet in height, and the flowers are whitish, tinged with purple. Patchouli first became known in Britain about 1820 when it was used to impregnate Indian shawls which became so fashionable that designs were copied by the Paisley weavers for export to many other parts of the world. They were unable to sell them, however, if not scented with patchouli. In the 1860s patchouli scents enjoyed the same popularity in England as they did in the 1960s. In the east the oil is used to scent linen, and the leaves are used in sachets and pot-pourris.

Patchouli oil has the unusual property of improving in odour with age. It is a deep reddish-brown, and is exactly the same colour and consistency as oils of benzoin and myrrh. The scent has been compared with the smell of goats, musty attics, and old coats. It has a very persistent odour, and is an excellent fixative; it is used in small quantities in rose, and oriental perfumes. It has a decidedly sour taste, indicating a possible use in disorders of the digestive process. It is patchouli and camphor that give Indian ink its characteristic smell.

Not a great deal is known about the therapeutic properties of patchouli oil. It has a fairly general but mild bactericidal action, is a notable aphrodisiac, and promotes the formation of scar tissue. It is one of the oils mentioned by Rovesti in connection with anxiety and depression, particularly the former. It is sometimes used in skin care products.

Although it is not hot and burning like mustard or pepper, patchouli gives the impression of being a very yang oil. It seems to be one of those oils that are stimulating in small doses, and sedative in large doses, like the sun. Its yang effect is most pronounced on the nervous system; it seems to be a very strong nerve stimulant, reminiscent of ginseng which, if you take enough, will help to keep you awake at night. Mrs Grieve mentions that patchouli sometimes causes loss of appetite and sleep. This is probably linked with its aphrodisiac effect, and, like ginseng, may involve an action on the endocrine glands. The effect of sedation or stimulation not only depends on the dose but also on the state of the individual.

The scent of patchouli recalls that of myrrh; they both have a kind of musty-sweet, heavy odour. Patchouli appears to have the astringent, antiphlogistic properties of myrrh; it has a very drying quality and is probably a good styptic. It binds, brings together, sharpens the wits, and is very good for mucousy, slow, phlegmatic types. It may be used for skin redness, weeping sores, and cracked skin. Mrs Grieve states that it contains 'coerulein', which probably refers to azulene, hence the antiphlogistic property.

Patchouli does not close up and obstruct where there is a natural flow, constricting only where there is abnormal looseness. In this it may be used as a tonic in diarrhoea, and constipation due to an enlarged, atonic colon. It may also prove useful in treating oedema, obesity, water retention, waterlogged skins, and perhaps the loose skin of the aged. In anxiety and depression its property may occasion a mild sedative effect, but more important, a bringing together of the thoughts, helping to clarify problems, and bring them to a point where they can be seen more objectively and dealt with.

Peppermint

Latin name	*Mentha piperita*
Family	*Labiatae*
Quality	Yang
Ruling planet	Mercury
Evaporation rate	70
Odour intensity	7
Essence from	Herb

Properties
Analgesic
Antiphlogistic
Antiseptic
Antispasmodic
Astringent
Carminative
Cephalic
Cholagogue
Cordial
Emmenagogue
Expectorant
Febrifuge
Hepatic
Nervine
Stomachic
Sudorific
Vasoconstrictor
Vermifuge

Uses
Asthma
Bronchitis
Cholera
Colds
Colic
Cough
Dermatitis
Diarrhoea
Dysmenorrhoea
Dyspepsia
Fainting
Fevers
Flatulence
Gall stones
Gastralgia
Halitosis
Headache
Hysteria

Influenza
Mental fatigue
Migraine
Nausea
Nervous disorders
Neuralgia
Palpitation
Paralysis
Pruritis
Ringworm
Scabies
Shock
Sinusitis
Toothache
Tuberculosis
Vertigo
Vomiting

Peppermint is one of the most important oils therapeutically, and is also widely used in commerce; in sweets, toothpastes, and so on. The plant was not distinguished from other mints until the seventeenth century. Pliny tells us that the Greeks and Romans crowned themselves with peppermint at their feasts, and that it was used to flavour both their sauces and their wines. It was used, along with other mints, by the ancient Greek physicians, and there is some evidence that it was even cultivated by the Egyptians.

It is cultivated in many parts of the world including Italy, the USA, Japan and Great Britain. The USA produces more oil than any other country, but the European oils are regarded as being superior in quality to any other.

It is a native of the Mediterranean, although Greek mythology offers a more romantic tale. Mint was once the nymph Mentha, whom Pluto found extremely attractive. Persephone, his jealous wife, pursued Mentha and trod her ferociously into the ground! Pluto then changed Mentha into a delightful herb.

'To promote the appetite when an impediment of the stomach cometh of cold humours being in the mouth of the stomach, make a sauce of mints and vinegar with a little cinnamon and pepper and use it well against vomits that come of feebleness of the stomach or of cold causes. Seethe mints in sage water and vinegar and dip it in and lay it on the mouth of the stomach with the mints that be sodden therein. Also, give to the patient to est of the same mints for the syncopyne [fainting] and feebleness in fevers and without fevers, either of medicine, or of what cause it be. Stamp mints with vinegar, and a little wine if the patient be without fever, and if he be with fever stamp mints with vinegar alone; then make a toast of sour bread and toast it well till it be almost burnt; then put it in that liquor and let it lie therein till it be well soaked; then put it into his nose and rub his lips, gums, teeth, and temples therewith and bind it to the pulse veins of his arms, and let the patient eat the moistness that is left and swallow it in. For to cleanse the mother [mother], take the tender crops of mints and seethe them in water or wine and plaster it to the share [pubes] and to the reins. Against the congealing in a woman's breasts, take the small stalks of mints

267

and seethe them in wine and oil and plaster it about the teats. Also, be it known that when any medicine should be given against venom, it should be given with the juice of mints, for mints have a manner of strength in drawing out of venom or else it should be given with wine that mints have been sodden in. For stopping of the spleen and the liver and of the ways of the urine by a cold humour and by a hot without fever, take the juice of mints alone or mints sodden in wine or the juice of mints meddles with honey and give it to the patient. To slay worms in the belly, take the juice of mints and drink it, and thou shall be whole' (Banckes's *Herbal*).

'This herb has a strong, agreeable, aromatic smell, and a moderate warm bitterish taste; it is useful for complaints of the stomach, such as wind, vomiting, etc. for which there are few remedies of greater efficacy. It is good in poultices and fomentations to disperse curdled milk in the breasts, and also to be used with milk diets. All mints are astringent, and of warm subtle parts; great strengtheners of the stomach. Their fragrance betokens them cephalics; they effectually take off nauseausness and retchings to vomit; they are also of use in looseness. The simple water given to children, removes the gripes' (Nicholas Culpeper).

'esteemed by some to be an excellent remedy against the stone and gravel' (Joseph Miller).

'These grateful aromatics [i.e. the essences of mints] are rapidly absorbed into the system, and behave as mild diffusible stimulants. Coming into contact with the gastric mucous membrane, they exercise at first a stimulating and afterwards a local sedative effect, dispelling nausea, and correcting uneasiness. By their local stimulating action on the bowel they correct the irregular painful sensations caused by accumulation of flatus, giving speedy relief, probably through a reflex act by driving on the imprisoned gas. Often after a large dose, pain instantly disappears, and flatus is expelled, and this may be frequently observed in infants and feeble females' (William Whitla).

Peppermint oil really needs no description, as its refreshing taste and odour is familiar to all. It is not easy to pin down the essential qualities of this oil since it has such a wide-ranging action; this is confirmed by its taste, which is a combination of sweet, bitter, and sour. Its most obvious quality when tasted, or applied to the skin, is that of cooling; and yet it is traditionally described as heating and drying. In fact the warming effect of peppermint is really the reaction of the body to a cold stimulus, and in this it strongly resembles camphor. It we look at menthol we find that it has the yin qualities of peppermint, but even more strongly. Menthol is its principal constituent, and is responsible for most of its therapeutic action.

Always use peppermint instead of aspirin.

For its analgesic, sedative, cooling effects to predominate fairly large and/or repeated doses of peppermint oil must be employed. It is good for disorders of both heat and cold, and so is ideal for most types of fever, colds, influenza, etc. Its action on the digestive system is most pronounced: it is the prime remedy for all digestive disorders including indigestion, colic, flatulence, stomach pains, diarrhoea (for which it is also a very good antiseptic). It is an effective remedy for nausea and vomiting; it relieves nausea almost instantaneously, and is good also for sea or travel sickness. For headaches and migraines related to digestive or hepatic phenomena it is an excellent remedy. In this connection it is also useful for skin disorders; it relieves internal toxic congestion, acts as a sudorific, and externally has an antiseptic/anti-inflammatory effect.

As a cooling, antiseptic, antispasmodic expectorant peppermint oil is very useful in respiratory disorders. It is a fairly good antibacterial agent in tuberculosis. It is very good for a dry cough. It is especially good for sinus congestion, infection, or inflammation, and for congestive headache. If you think too much, or have a hot head, it will cool you down. If you feel faint it will stabilise your head and dispel nausea. As an analgesic-emmenagogue it is very good for dysmenorrhoea and also for scanty menstruation. Applied externally it relieves the breast of curdled or congested milk, and prevents infection. Internally it will discourage the flow of milk to the breast. It strengthens and numbs the nerves, and in large doses will put you to sleep. It is valuable in many nervous disorders such as hysteria, palpitations, trembling, and paralysis. It helps to break up gall stones, and may also be good for kidney stones. The Menominees, a tribe of North American Indians, used peppermint leaves to treat pneumonia. It has also been used to treat anaemia.

Peppermint oil will relieve any kind of skin irritation or itching, but should be used in moderation (less than 1%) or the irritation will be made worse. It may be used for skin redness due to inflammation, or acne; it cools by constricting the capillaries, and is a very refreshing skin tonic. Peppermint is effective against ringworm and scabies, and is used in homeopathy for shingles. It makes a very invigorating and refreshing bath oil, which helps to cool down the body in summertime. It is a mosquito and rat repellent.

Rose

Latin name	*Rosa damascena* (Damask rose)
	Rosa centifolia (cabbage rose)
Family	Rosaceae
Quality	Yin
Ruling planet	Venus
Evaporation rate	99
Odour intensity	7
Essence from	Flowers

Properties
Antidepressant
Antiphlogistic
Antiseptic
Antispasmodic
Aphrodisiac
Astringent
Choleretic
Depurative
Emmenagogue
Haemostatic
Hepatic
Laxative
Sedative
Splenetic
Stomachic
Tonic (heart,
  stomach, liver,
  uterus)

Uses
Cholecystitis
Conjunctivitis
Constipation
Depression
Frigidity
Haemorrhage
Headache
Hepatic congestion
Impotence
Insomnia
Irregular
  menstruation
Leucorrhoea
Menorrhagia
Nausea
Nervous tension
Ophthalmia
Skin care

Sterility
Uterine disorders
Vomiting

'The rose distils a healing balm
the beating pulse of pain to calm' (Anacreon).

If jasmine is king of all aromatics, then rose is certainly queen. There is something unmistakably feminine about the scent of roses, and one of their main medicinal uses is for what are vaguely termed 'female complaints'. The rose is said to have sprung up from the blood of Adonis, while Gerarde tells us that the Turks believe it sprang from the blood of Venus, and the Mohammedans that it sprang from the sweat of Mohamet.

Roses have been used for their appearance, their scent, and their therapeutic properties from time immemorial. They were used extensively by the Romans for garlands, perfumes, scented baths, confections, and as a remedy for hangover.

Rose oil itself was said to be accidentally discovered in Persia at the wedding fest of the princess Nour-Djihan and the Emperor Djihanguyr. A canal was dug, encircling the gardens, and it was filled with rose water. The heat of the sun caused the oil to separate and float to the top where it was noticed as a kind of scum. When this 'scum' was examined, and its true nature discovered, it was not long before the production of Persian rose oil began.

The rose was used to adorn the shields of Persian warriors at the time of their supremacy and, according to Ibn Khaldun, the province of Farnistan provided an annual tribute of 30,000 bottles of rose water to the treasury at Baghdad.

The production of Persian rose oil, like that of India, is no longer large enough to be commercially significant. The finest and most expensive rose oil comes from Bulgaria, and is known as Bulgarian rose otto. It is extracted from the damask rose, which can only be successfully cultivated in a mountainous district approximately 240 square miles in area and 1,300 feet above sea-level. From this plant, which is also cultivated in both Turkey and Morocco, an absolute and an otto are produced. Rose de mai (*Rosa centifolia*) is cultivated in the Grasse region of southern France, but it is only used for the production of an absolute, not an otto.

The colour of rose oil is orange/green, not red, as one would have thought. It takes 30 roses to make one drop of Bulgarian rose otto, and 60,000 roses (about 180 lb) to make one ounce.

Banckes's *Herbal* contains recipes for mell roset (rose honey), sugar roset, syrup of roses, an electuary of roses, water of roses, and oil of roses. He devotes more space to the rose than any other herb in the book, and some of his comments are reproduced here:

'This is the red rose. It is cold in the first degree and dry in the second degree . . . Some stamp fresh roses with oil, and they put it in a vessel of glass and set in the sun fifty days, and this oil is good against the chafing of the liver, if it be anointed therewith. Also it is good for the disease in the head that cometh of heat: anoint the forehead and the temples with oil of roses. The water of roses hath virtue of comforting and constraining against the flux of the womb and the vomit . . . Also, rose water is good for the Syncopyne and the cardiacle: give it him to drink and sprinkle the water on his face. Also, the water is good for eyes and in ointments for the face, for it taketh away the wems [blemishes] and the superfluity and straineth the skin. Also, dry roses put the nose to smell do comfort the brain and the heart and quickeneth the spirit.'

Gerarde tells us that rose water 'mitigateth the paine of the eies proceeding of the hot cause, bringeth sleep which also the fresh roses themselves provoke through their sweet and pleasant smell'.
Culpeper has some interesting things to say about roses:

'The damask rose, on account of its fragrance, belongs to the cephaltics; but the next valuable virtue it possesses, consists in its cathartic quality.
'The flowers of the common red rose dried, are given in infusions, and sometimes in powder, against overflowing of the menses, spitting of blood, and other haemorrhages.'

He also mentions that red rose tincture is good for strengthening the stomach, and preventing vomiting.

'The white and red roses are cooling and drying . . . The decoction of red roses made with wine and used, is very good for head-ache, and pains in the eyes, ears, throat and gums; as also for the fundament and the lower parts of the belly and the matrix, being bathed or put into them. The same decoction . . . is applied to the region of the heart, to ease the inflammation therein . . .

273

'Red roses strengthen the heart, the stomach, the liver and the retentive faculty; they mitigate the pains that arise from heat, cool inflammations, procure rest and sleep . . .

'Oil of roses is used by itself to cool hot inflammation or swellings, and to bind and stay fluxes of humours to sores.'

Joseph Miller writes about all three types of rose. The white rose is 'drying, binding and cooling'. Of damask rose, he says: 'The flowers are of a gentle cathartic nature, purging choleric and serous humours, being given to children and weakly persons, and mixt frequently with stronger cathartics.' The red rose 'is more binding and restringent than any of the other species, good against all kinds of fluxes; they strengthen the stomach, prevent vomiting, and stop tickling coughs, by preventing the defluxion of rheum, and are of great service in consumptions'.

Dr Chandrashekhar has this to say:

'The rose is cooling, soothing, and beneficial to the heart and eyes. It is a laxative, and a tonic; and increases semen, and enhances beauty of the complexion. It has a combined bitter and sweet taste. It is a digestive, restores the balance of tridoshas [primary qualities] and it is highly efficacious in blood impurities.'

Li Shih-Chên tells us of a highly fragrant rose, *Rosa rugosa*, which is cultivated in China:

'Its nature is cooling, its taste is sweet with a slight bitterishness, and it acts especially on the spleen and liver, promoting the circulation of the blood. It is prescribed in the form of an extract for haematemesis, and the flowers are used in all diseases of the liver, to scatter abcesses, and in blood diseases generally . . . Essence of Rose is made by distilling the flowers of Rosa rugosa. Its medicinal action is upon the liver, stomach, and blood. It drives away melancholy.'

He also mentions essence of *Rosa indica*: 'It is used as a heart remedy and in the treatment of melancholy.'

Marguerite Maury wrote:

> 'As a well-known aphrodisiac, it is used in the Hindu pharmacopoeia reinforced with sandalwood. Our own experiences have taught us that the rose has a considerable influence on the female sexual organs. Not by stimulus, but on the contrary, by cleansing and regulating their functions. We have been able to test its influence on cardiac rhythm and blood circulation. The capillaries — those little hearts with independent beats — become active once more, and capillaropathy, with its sometimes tragic consequences, can be perfectly cured.'

The Mescalero Apaches boiled wild rosebuds and imbibed the resulting tea to treat gonorrhoea.

These quotations speak eloquently for themselves. But to summarise, rose tones the vascular and digestive systems through a purging, cleansing action rather than a stimulating one. It also has a soothing action on the nerves, which may induce sleep, although it is not a strong sedative. Because of its excellent fragrance it can also be regarded as an anti-depressant. It is a known aphrodisiac, is said to increase semen, and may well be of use in cases of impotence or sterility. Being ruled by Venus it is of great use in regulating the menstrual function, is a gentle emmenagogue, and cleanses the womb of impurities. It may be used in all disorders of the genito-urinary system. Its action on the vascular system is manifold: it promotes the circulation, cleanses the blood relieves cardiac congestion, regulates the action of spleen and heart, and tones the capillaries. Its action on the digestive system is almost as important; it strengthens the stomach, promotes the flow of bile, and the elimination of faeces. It is also useful for nausea, vomiting, and coughing or vomiting blood. The external use of rose water on the eyes reduces inflammation, and is of use in conjunctivitis.

The triple action of rose on the vascular, digestive, and nervous systems, and more especially the nature of its action, render it particularly suitable for the conditions of stress which are becoming more and more common today: nervous tension, peptic ulcers, heart disease, and so on.

Modern research has little to add to what Culpeper and his contemporaries already knew about the rose. In 1972 a paper was published in the USSR on the choleretic action of rose oil. The addition of rose oil to the food of rats was found to increase the secretion of bile fluid and major organic components of bile. The conclusion is drawn that rose oil may stimulate hepatic bile formation in humans, especially the synthesis of bile acids and phospholipids. It may be useful in the treatment of cholecystitis, and perhaps of jaundice.

Rose oil is, perhaps surprisingly, one of the most antiseptic essences. This, combined with its slightly tonic and soothing qualities and its action on the capillaries, make it useful for virtually all types of skin. It is particularly good for mature, dry, or sensitive skin, and for any kind of redness, or inflammation.

Rose is the least toxic of all essences. For most therapeutic purposes, especially if it is being taken internally the essence, or otto, should be used in preference to the absolute.

Rosemary

Latin name	*Rosmarinus officinalis*
Family	*Labiatae*
Quality	Yang
Ruling planet	Sun
Evaporation rate	18
Odour intensity	6
Essence from	Herb

Properties

Adrenal cortex
  stimulant
Analgesic
Antiseptic
Antispasmodic
Astringent
Carminative
Cephalic
Cholagogue
Choleretic
Cicatrisant
Cordial
Digestive
Diuretic
Emmenagogue
Hepatic
Hypertensor
Nervine
Stimulant
Stomachic
Sudorific
Vulnerary

Uses

Asthma
Arteriosclerosis
Baldness
Bronchitis
Chlorosis
Cholecystitis
Cirrhosis
Colds
Colitis
Debility
Diarrhoea
Dysmenorrhoea
Dyspepsia
Epilepsy
Fainting
Flatulence
Gall stones
Gout
Headache
Hepatic disorders

Hypercholesterol-
  aemia
Hypotension
Hysteria
Influenza
Jaundice
Leucorrhoea
Mental fatigue
Migraine
Nervous disorders
Palpitations
Pediculosis
Phthisis
Rheumatism
Scabies
Skin care
Whooping cough
Wounds

Rosemary is one of the earliest and most renowned of the English medicinal herbs, although it is apparently not a native of this country. The ancients often used sprigs of rosemary to drive away evil spirits, and to burn as incense; an old French name for it is *incensier*. In France it was traditionally used to burn as a fumigant in sick rooms. It was used to flavour ale and wine, was put in with clothes to keep moths away, and was even used as a Christmas decoration. Like rue, it was placed in the dock of courts of justice to prevent the spreading of jail fever. It was commonly found in herb gardens, and was used as a condiment. It was medicinally used to strengthen the memory and nerves and to warm the heart.

Rosemary water was used as a beautifying and cleansing facial wash. It was also one of the main ingredients of Hungary water, which was named after Queen Elizabeth of Hungary, who used it as a rejuvenating lotion, washing her face with it every day. It is also reputed to have been used as a remedy for gout and paralysed limbs. Rosemary is also one of the ingredients of the classic Eau-de-Cologne, which will often relieve a headache when applied to the temples. In the sixth century Charlemagne decreed that rosemary should be grown in all the imperial gardens.

The name of rosemary comes from the Latin *ros marinus*, meaning sea dew, as it is fond of water. It is a well-known perennial herb with long, straight stems studded with one-inch long narrow, pointed leaves. These are deep green on the upper side and silvery grey underneath. It grows up to some six feet in height, and has small, pale blue flowers.

Rosemary oil is clear and has a warm, sharp, camphoraceous taste which has, surprisingly, very little bitterness. Its similarity to camphor is very noticeable. It blends well with other fresh scents, like bergamot, basil, and peppermint, and makes an invigorating and refreshing bath oil.

'Rosemary. For weyknesse of ye brayne. Agaynst weyknesse of the brayne and coldeness thereof, sethe rosmarin in wyne and lete the pacyent receye the smoke at his nose and kepe his heed warme' (*The Grete Herball*).

'This herb is hot and dry . . . Also, take the flowers and make powder thereof and bind it to the right arm

in a linen cloth, and it shall make thee light and merry
. . . Also, boil the flowers in goat's milk and then let
them stand all a night under the air, fair covered;
after that give him to drink thereof that hath the
phthisic, and it shall deliver him. Also, boil the leaves
in white wine and wash thy face therewith, thy beard
and thy brows, and there shall no corns grow out, but
thou shall have a fair face. Also, but the leaves under
thy bed's head, and thou shall be delivered of all evil
dreams . . .

'Also, if thou have the flux, boil the leaves in
strong eisell and then bind them in a linen cloth and
bind it to thy womb, and anon the flux shall
withdraw. Also, if thy legs be blown with the gout,
boil the leaves in water and then take the leaves and
bind them in a linen cloth about thy legs, and it shall
do thee much good. Also, take the leaves and boil
them in a strong eisell and bind them in a cloth to thy
stomach, and it shall deliver thee of all evils'
(Banckes's *Herbal*).

'The Arabians and other Physitions succeeding, do
write, that Rosemary comforteth the braine, the
memorie, the inward senses, and restoreth speech unto
them that are possessed with the dumbe palsie,
especially the conserve made of the floures and sugar,
or any other way confected with sugar, being taken
every day fasting.

'The floures made up into plates with Sugar after
the manner of Sugar Roset and eaten, comfort the
heart, and make it merry, quicken the spirits, and
make them more lively' (John Gerarde).

'The decoction of Rosemary in wine, helps the cold
distillations of rheums into the eyes, and other cold
diseases of the head and brain, as the giddiness and
swimmings therein, drowsiness of dulness, the dumb
palsy, or loss of speech, the lethargy, the falling-
sickness, to be both drunk and the temples bathed
therewith . . . It helps a weak memory and quickens
the senses.

'The chymical [essential] oil drawn from the leaves

and flowers, is a sovereign help for all the diseases aforesaid, to touch the temples and nostrils with two or three drops for all the diseases of the head and brain spoken of before; as also to take one drop, two or three, as the case requires, for the inward diseases; yet it must be done with discretion, for it is very quick and piercing, and therefore but a little must be taken at a time' (Nicholas Culpeper).

By the turn of the eighteenth century rosemary oil was an official preparation. It is a yang oil, and is very piercing, and stimulating; it stings like basil, only to a lesser degree, and does not burn like mustard or pepper. Its stimulating nature has led to its use in loss of the sense of smell, and in loss of speech, although its efficacy here obviously depends on the cause of the condition. It is also recommended for 'dim eyes' by Culpeper, who says that it 'procures a clear sight'. It is ruled by the sun, and has a warming, stimulating effect on the heart. It has a similar effect on the mind and the nerves, and has also been traditionally used for loss of memory, vertigo, and general dullness.

Rosemary oil is a very good nerve stimulant, and may be used in all disorders where there is a reduction or loss of nerve function. In the case of sensory nerves this may result in impaired sensual perception, and in the case of motor nerves in paralysis, loss of speech, etc. It is also of value in most other nervous disorders, including hysteria and epilepsy. Rosemary is a valuable stimulant where there is general sluggishness, debility, or apathy, and it normalises low blood pressure. It also has a pronounced action on the brain, similar to that of basil; it will clear the mind of confusion and doubt, and is a classic remedy for fainting, headache, and migraine.

It is an excellent heart tonic, having a mild stimulating action, and is good for nervous cardiac disorders, such as palpitations. It is also good for many liver disorders, including chlorosis, hepatism, cirrhosis, and as a cholagogue may be used in cholecystitis, gall stones, and jaundice due to hepatitis or bile duct blockage. Rosemary oil helps to normalise a high cholesterol level in the blood, hence its use in arteriosclerosis.

The antiseptic action of rosemary is especially suitable for intestinal infection and diarrhoea. Its action on the digestion is stimulating, antispasmodic, carminative, and stomachic. It may be used for colitis, atonic dyspepsia, flatulence, and stomach pains.

As an antispasmodic rosemary may be used in asthma and chronic bronchitis; as an antiseptic, warming oil it is useful in colds, influenza, and associated coughs. Being under the rulership of the sun rosemary is very good for wasting diseases; Culpeper comments: 'The dried leaves shred small, and smoked as tobacco, helps those that have any cough, phthisis, or consumption, by warming and drying the thin distillations which cause those diseases.'

Applied externally rosemary oil is very good for rheumatic or muscular pain, and may be used as a general remedy for gout and rheumatism. It is good for lice and scabies, and is an excellent wound remedy. The Arabs sprinkle the powdered herb on the umbilical cord of new-born infants as an astringent antiseptic. The use of rosemary oil in scalp disorders is traditional. It is stimulating and cleansing, and is very good for loss of hair or dandruff. In skin care rosemary may be used as a tonic-astringent, especially in the form of an aromatic water.

Sandalwood

Latin name	*Santalum album*
Family	*Santalaceae*
Quality	Yang
Ruling planet	Uranus
Evaporation rate	100?
Odour intensity	5
Essence from	Wood

Properties
Antidepressant
Antiphlogistic
Antiseptic
Antispasmodic
Aphrodisiac
Astringent
Carminative
Diuretic
Expectorant
Sedative
Tonic

Uses
Acne
Blenorrhoea
Bronchitis
Catarrh
Cough
Cystitis
Depression
Diarrhoea
Gonorrhoea
Hiccough
Insomnia
Laryngitis
Nausea
Nervous tension
Skin care
Tuberculosis
Vomiting

The sandalwood tree grows to a height of twenty to thirty feet, and has red, yellow, or violet/pink flowers. Only the inner wood, known as the heart-wood, is used. Sandalwood has been used from earliest times as incense, in embalming, and in cosmetics. In ancient India it was widely used in religious ceremonies, and was regarded as a panacea, although they also recognised its specific value in genito-urinary affections. It is mentioned in the *Nirukta*, the oldest Vedic commentary known, which was written during the fifth century BC. In India and Egypt it was used as a perfume, and was an ingredient of many cosmetics. The Chinese used to import it, and employed it in similar ways; they now grow their own. A variety of curios, furniture, and other wooden articles are still made from sandalwood in the East. Because sandalwood is one of the few woods immune to attack by white ants it used to be widely used in building. This, however, led to a great number of trees being cut down. All sandalwood trees are now the property of the Indian Government, and most of the wood is used to distil the essence. The name sandalwood is probably derived from the Sanskrit *chandana*.

Santalum album grows in East India (Mysore) and the Lingnan region of China. The Chinese oil is not commercially available. West Indian sandalwood, which is known as amyris oil, comes from a completely different species, *Schimmelia oleifera*. Its scent is distinctly inferior to Mysore sandalwood, and its therapeutic properties are little known. There is also Australian sandalwood oil, which is distilled from *Santalum spicatum*. This is closer to Mysore sandalwood both botanically and odoriferously, and it is used medicinally. Its therapeutic properties do not generally come up to the standard of the Mysore oil.

Sandalwood oil has been used more than any other essence as a perfume in its own right. It is also a valuable fixative, and is widely used in high-class perfumes. The scent is woody, sweet, reminiscent of rose, with a spicy, oriental undertone. It blends well with most other oils, especially rose, orange blossom, and benzoin. It has a thick, oily consistency, and a faint greenish-yellow colour. The taste is extremely bitter. This is quite interesting, because the back part of the tongue, which registers bitter tastes, is supplied by a branch of the vagus nerve. The vagus, or tenth cranial nerve, supplies the pharynx, larynx, lungs, heart, gall bladder, and stomach. Bitter tonics are used in herbal medicine to stimulate digestion. Sandalwood has a very pronounced action on the mucous membranes of the genito-urinary and pulmonary tracts, and is often used in chronic infections of these areas. It is effective against streptococcus and staphylococcus aureus and so is suitable for most types of sore throat, including laryngitis. Its expectorant and antispasmodic properties are also very useful in chronic bronchitis and coughs. It is effective against the avian type of mycobacterium tuberculosis. It should be used in all pulmonary conditions where there is catarrh, and will also relieve a dry cough.

Sandalwood oil is effective in all genito-urinary conditions where there is a mucousy discharge, especially gonorrhoea. It does not exert a definite bactericidal effect in gonococcal infection, but is of value in that it abolishes spontaneous contractions of the spermatic cord, lessens the motility of the genital tract muscles, has a diuretic effect, and inhibits secretions. It is more of a male remedy, but may also be used in leucorrhoea. It has an anti-inflammatory and mild analgesic effect in inflammation of the mucous membrane.

Li Shih-Chên recommends sandalwood for hiccough, vomiting, choleraic difficulties, and acne. The oil relieves intestinal spasm and inflammation, and may be useful in colic and gastritis. It is of great value in both acute and chronic diarrhoea. From its very bitter taste, and a possible reflex action via the vagus nerve, sandalwood may be useful in aiding digestion, and may have a specific action on the gall bladder. This is supported by Li Shis-Chên's 'choleraic difficulties'.

Sandalwood is a mild, yang oil. It is emollient, tonic, sedative, and very useful in chronic and inflammatory disorders. Because of its agreeable scent it may be of use in states of anxiety and depression; being quite a heavy oil it is more sedative than uplifting. From its action on the vagus nerve, it would seem likely to have a sedative, tonic, antispasmodic effect on the heart, which would be serviceable in states of nervous tension. Mme Maury writes: 'Rose and sandalwood oil compensate for renal and cardiac deficiencies', although she may only be referring to sandalwood for its effects on the kidneys. In oriental medicine a bitter taste is associated with the heart and small intestine.

Oil of sandalwood is one of the most useful oils for the skin. It is the classic choice for dry skin, and for dehydrated skin should be applied with warm compresses. It relieves itching and inflammation of the skin, and acts as an antiseptic in acne. As a mild astringent it may be profitably used in oily skin conditions. No wonder the ancients valued it as a cosmetic!

Ylang-ylang

Latin name	*Cananga odorata*
Family	*Anonaceae*
Quality	Yin
Ruling planet	Venus
Evaporation rate	91
Odour intensity	6
Essence from	Flowers

Properties
Antidepressant
Antiseptic
Aphrodisiac
Hypotensor
Sedative

Uses
Depression
Frigidity
Hyperpnoea
Hypertension
Impotence

Insomnia
Nervous tension
Palpitations
Skin care

The ylang-ylang tree grows to a height of sixty feet, and has beautiful yellow flowers. It is cultivated in Java, Sumatra, Réunion, Madagascar, and the Comores; the finest oil used to come from the Philippines, but unfortunately this is no longer obtainabie. Ylang-ylang should not be confused with 'cananga oil', which is an inferior product. It has been suggested that cananga and ylang-ylang are the same plant, but its cultivation in different parts of the world produces slight differences in the essential oil.

Its name means flower of flowers, and it certainly has an exotic, voluptuous scent. It resembles a mixture of jasmine and almond, and is very sweet. It blends well with sandalwood and jasmine, and makes a useful fixative. The oil has a slight yellow tint, and a fairly bland taste, slightly bitter and slightly sweet; it forms an ingredient of the famous Macassar hair oil. R. W. Moncrieff in his book on *Odours* comments:

'The effects of some odours on the emotions are quite strong. The writer, working with odorous materials

for more than twenty years, long ago noticed that . . .
ylang-ylang oil soothes and inhibits anger born of
frustration.'

Ylang-ylang is one of the most pleasant oils, and may readily
be used as a lasting perfume and an exotic bath oil. Its effect on
the nervous system is euphoric, sedative, hypotensive, and it is
indicated in states of anxiety, tension, and high blood pressure.
It is a very good aphrodisiac, and may be of use in impotence or
frigidity. As well as reducing high blood pressure it relieves
tachycardia (abnormally fast heart-beat) and hyperpnoea (abor-
mally fast breathing).

As a general antiseptic it is of moderate value, but is particularly useful for intestinal infections. It has a soothing effect
on the skin, and is widely used in facial massage oils because of
its scent. It is also reputed to be good for oily types of skin.

Do not use ylang-ylang in concentrated amounts; it has a
strong, sweet odour, and too much will only cause headache or
nausea.

Table I

Essential oil	Odour intensity	Evaporation rate	Quality	Ruling planet
Basil	7	78	Yang	Mars
Benzoin	4	100?	Yang	Sun
Bergamot	4	55	Yang	Sun
Black pepper	7	60	Yang	Mars
Camomile	9	47	Yin	Moon
Camphor	5	?	Yin	Saturn
Cardamon	9	68	Yang	Mercury
Cedarwood	4	97	Yang	Jupiter
Clary sage	5	82	Yang	Mercury
Cypress	4	30	Yin	Saturn
Eucalyptus	8	5	Yin	Saturn
Fennel	6	85	Yang	Mercury
Frankincense	7	75	Yang	Sun
Geranium	6	87	Yin	Venus
Hyssop	6	65	Yang	Jupiter
Jasmine	7	95	Yang	Jupiter
Juniper	5	30	Yang	Jupiter
Lavender	4	85	Yang	Mercury
Marjoram	5	40	Yang	Mercury
Melissa	4?	17	Yang	Jupiter
Myrrh	7	100?	Yang	Sun
Neroli	5	79	Yang	Sun
Patchouli	5	100	Yang	Sun
Peppermint	7	70	Yang	Mercury
Rose	7	99	Yin	Venus
Rosemary	6	18	Yang	Sun
Sandalwood	5	100?	Yang	Uranus
Ylang-ylang	6	91	Yin	Venus

Table II

Essence	Latin Name	Family
Basil	*Ocymum basilicum*	*Labiatae*
Benzoin	*Styrax benzoin*	*Styraceae*
Bergamot	*Citrus bergamia*	*Rutaceae*
Black pepper	*Piper nigrum*	*Piperaceae*
Camomile	*Anthemis nobilis*	*Compositae*
	Matricaria chamomilla	*Compositae*
Camphor	*Cinnamomum camphora*	*Lauraceae*
Cardamon	*Elettaria cardamomum*	*Zingiberaceae*
Cedarwood	*Juniperus virginiana*	*Coniferae*
Clary sage	*Salvia sclarea*	*Labiatae*
Cypress	*Cupressus sempervirens*	*Coniferae*
Eucalyptus	*Eucalyptus globulus*	*Myrtaceae*
Fennel	*Foeniculum vulgare*	*Umbelliferae*
Frankincense	*Boswellia thurifera*	*Burseraceae*
Geranium	*Pelargonium odorantissimum*	*Geraniaceae*
	Pelargonium graveolens	*Geraniaceae*
Hyssop	*Hyssopus officinalis*	*Labiatae*
Jasmine	*Jasminum officinale*	*Jasminaceae*
	Jasminum grandiflorum	*Jasminaceae*
Juniper	*Juniperus communis*	*Coniferae*
Lavender	*Lavandula officinalis*	*Labiatae*
	Lavandula angustifolia	*Labiatae*
Marjoram	*Origanum marjorana*	*Labiatae*
Melissa	*Melissa officinalis*	*Labiatae*
Myrrh	*Commiphora myrrha*	*Burseraceae*
	Balsamodendron myrrha	*Burseraceae*
Neroli	*Citrus aurantium*	*Rutaceae*
Patchouli	*Pogostemon patchouli*	*Labiatae*
Peppermint	*Mentha piperita*	*Labiatae*
Rose	*Rose centifolia*	*Rosaceae*
	Rosa damascena	*Rosaceae*
Rosemary	*Rosmarinus officinalis*	*Labiatae*
Sandalwood	*Santalum album*	*Santalaceae*
Ylang-ylang	*Cananga odorata*	*Anonaceae*

Table III

Odour Intensity Index

4	Benzoin		7	Basil
	Bergamot			Black pepper
	Cedarwood			Frankincense
	Cypress			Jasmine
	Lavender			Myrrh
	Melissa?			Peppermint
				Rose

5	Camphor
	Clary sage
	Juniper
	Marjoram
	Neroli
	Patchouli
	Sandalwood

8	Eucalyptus
9	Camomile
	Cardamon

6	Fennel	Rosemary
	Geranium	Ylang-ylang
	Hyssop	

Table IV

Volatility Index

5	Eucalyptus	82	Clary sage
18	Rosemary	85	Fennel
30	Cypress	85	Lavender
30	Juniper	87	Geranium
40	Marjoram	91	Ylang-ylang
47	Camomile	95	Jasmine
55	Bergamot	97	Cedarwood
60	Black pepper	99	Rose
65	Hyssop	100	Patchouli
68	Cardamon	100	Benzoin?
70	Peppermint	100	Myrrh?
75	Frankincense	100	Sandalwood?
78	Basil		
79	Neroli		

Table V

Evaporation Rates

(Poucher)

3	Myrrh	21	Rosemary
4	Eucalyptus Lavender	24	Ylang-ylang
		29	Geranium
6	Bergamot	30	Cardamon
8	Cedarwood Rose (centifolia)	40	Hyssop
9	Peppermint	43	Jasmine Rose (gallica)
10	Camomile	50	Neroli
14	Basil Fennel	100	Benzoin Black pepper Cypress Frankincense Patchouli Sandalwood
15	Rose (damask)		
17	Melissa		
18	Marjoram		
20	Clary sage		

Numbers 1 – 14 are considered as top notes,
15 – 60 are middle notes, and
61 – 100 are base notes.

Table VI

Yang and Yin Oils

Yang Oils		Yin Oils	
Mercury (Air)	Cardamom	*Venus* (Earth)	Geranium
	Clary sage		Rose
	Fennel		Ylang-ylang
	Lavender		
	Marjoram	*Saturn* (Earth)	Camphor
	Peppermint		Cypress
			Eucalyptus
Uranus (Air)	Cedarwood		
	Sandalwood	*Moon* (Water)	Camomile
Jupiter (Fire)	Hyssop		
	Jasmine		
	Juniper		
	Melissa		
Sun (Fire)	Benzoin		
	Bergamot		
	Frankincense		
	Myrrh		
	Neroli		
	Patchouli		
	Rosemary		
Mars (Fire)	Basil		
	Black pepper		

Some Complementary Relationships of Yin and Yang

YIN	YANG
Female	Male
Passive	Active
Inwards	Outwards
Contracts	Expands
Closing	Opening
Emptiness	Fullness
Dark	Light
Cold	Hot
Moist	Dry
Sedative	Stimulant
Inhalation	Exhalation
Venous blood	Arterial blood
Parasympathetic nerves	Sympathetic nerves
Fear	Anger
Caution	Courage
Blue	Red

Glossary of Medical Terms

Acetylcholine	a fluid which transmits messages from one nerve ending to another
Albuminuria	presence of albumin in the urine
Alopecia	baldness
Amenorrhoea	absence of menstruation
Aphthae	small white spots, in the mouth, caused by fungus
Arteriosclerosis	hardening of the arteries
Ataraxia	peace of mind
Auricular	refers to the upper chambers of the heart
Blenorrhoea	mucus discharge from the genitals
Blepharitis	inflammation of the eyelids
Cellulitis	'orange peel skin' caused by local accumulations of fat and toxic matter
Chlorosis	a form of anaemia
Cholecystitis	inflammation of the gall bladder
Cicatrisation	formation of scar tissue
Cirrhosis	chronic inflammation (most commonly of the liver)
Cutaneous	pertaining to the skin
Dropsy	abnormal accumulation of fluid in a body cavity
Dysmenorrhoea	painful menstruation
Dyspnoea	shortness of breath
Dysuria	difficulty or pain in passing water

Emphysema	a degerative disease of the lungs, in which the air sacs become abnormally enlarged
Endocrine	pertaining to ductless glands
Enuresis	the involuntary passing of urine
Erethism	an abnormal state of excitement or irritation
Exocrine	pertaining to a gland that secretes through a duct
Fibrillation	rapid twitching of muscle fibres
Fistula	an abnormal channel leading from a natural cavity to the exterior
Gingivitis	inflammation of the gums
Glomeronephritis	a form of nephritis, similar to Bright's disease
Glossitis	inflammation of the tongue
Haematuria	the presence of blood in the urine
Halitosis	offensive breath
Herpes	a vesicular eruption of the skin
Hypercholesterolaemia	excessive cholesterol in the blood
Hyperglycaemia	excess of sugar in the blood
Hyperpnoea	abnormally deep and rapid breathing
Hypertension	high blood pressure
Hypophyseal	pertaining to the pituitary gland
Hypotension	abnormally low blood pressure
Hysteria	abnormal state of mind characterised by exaggerated behaviour and physical disturbances
In vitro	in a test tube
In vivo	in a living body
Leucocytosis	the formation in the body of leucocytes (white blood cells)
Leucorrhoea	a whitish vaginal discharge
Menorrhagia	excessive loss of blood during menstruation
Nephritis	inflammation of the kidney
Neurasthenia	nervous exhaustion
Oedema	an excess of fluid beneath the skin
Olfaction	the sense of smell
Oliguria	low output of urine
Ophthalmia	inflammation of the eye

Otitis	inflammation of the ear
Parturient	aiding and easing childbirth
Phagocytosis	the absorbtion of foreign bodies by white blood cells
Pharmacopoeia	official book of drugs in common use
Polypus	a kind of growth (non-malignant)
Potentisation	a term used in homoeopathy to describe the diluting and succussion of a substance to release its energy
Prophylactic	preventative
Psoriasis	a chronic skin disease
Psychosomatic	pertaining to the mind and body
Pyelitis	inflammation of the pelvis of the kidney
Pyorrhoea	a discharge of pus, of the gums
Pyrosis	heartburn
Quinsy	large abscess of the throat
Scrofula	tuberculosis of the lymphatic glands
Spermatorrhoea	involuntary emission of semen without orgasm
Stomatitis	inflammation of the mucous membrane of the mouth
Strangury	painful or difficult passing of urine
Syphilid	A form of skin syphilis
Tic	a repetitive twitching
Urticaria	weals in the skin; also known as nettle rash

Terms used by the old herbalists

Ague	intermittent fever
Cast	vomit
Catamenia	menstruation
Cephalic	relating to the head, especially the brain
Courses	periods
Distemper	ailment
Eisell	vinegar
Falling sickness	epilepsy
Flux	watery discharge. May refer to blood, mucus, urine, etc., or body fluids in general

Megrim, migram	migraine
Palsy	paralysis
Reins	kidneys
Rheum	watery secretion. Usually refers to saliva or mucus, as in colds
Secundines	afterbirth
Seethe	steep, soak
Syncopyne	fainting
Yellow evil	jaundice

Therapeutic Index

Abscess	bergamot, lavender
Acne	
local:	bergamot, camphor, cedarwood, juniper, lavender, sandalwood
general:	non-toxic diet and depurative essences
Albuminuria	juniper
Alcoholism	fennel rose (see also *liver*, cirrhosis)
Allergies	camomile, melissa
Alopecia	lavender, rosemary
Amenorrhoea	see *menstruation*
Anaemia	camomile
Anxiety	see *nervous tension*
Aphthae	geranium, myrrh
Appendicitis	(first-aid only) lavender compresses
Appetite (loss of)	ascertain cause, and treat accordingly. A fast is probably indicated. Many essences stimulate appetite, including camomile, cardamon, fennel
Arteriosclerosis	juniper, rosemary
Arteritis	marjoram
Arthritis	see *rheumatism*
Asthma	benzoin, cypress, eucalyptus, hyssop, lavender, marjoram, melissa
Baldness	see *alopecia*

Blenorrhoea bergamot, cedarwood, eucalyptus, frankincense, juniper, lavender, sandalwood

Blepharitis see *conjunctivitis*

Boils
local: camomile, clary, lavender
general: non-toxic diet, depurative essences

Breasts
insufficient milk (of nursing mothers): fennel, jasmine
engorgement: geranium, peppermint

Bronchitis basil, benzoin, bergamot, camphor, cardamon, cedarwood, eucalyptus, frankincense, hyssop, lavender, peppermint, rosemary, sandalwood

Bruises camphor, hyssop

Burns
local: camomile, camphor, eucalpytus, geranium, lavender
general: see *shock*

Cancer
general: cedarwood? cypress? eucalyptus, hyssop
uterine cancer: bergamot, eucalyptus, geranium (these essences are not put forward as complete cures in themselves)

Carbuncles
local: bergamot, frankincense, lavender
general: non-toxic diet, depurative essences

Catarrh cedarwood, eucalyptus, frankincense, hyssop, lavender, myrrh, sandalwood

Cellulitis
local: juniper, lavender, rosemary
general: non-toxic diet

Childbirth jasmine, lavender

Chlorosis see *liver*

Cholecystitis see *gall bladder*

Cholera black pepper, camphor, eucalyptus, peppermint

Circulation
hypertension: clary, hyssop, lavender, marjoram, melissa, ylang-ylang
hypotension: camphor, hyssop, rosemary
Cirrhosis   see *liver*
Colds   basil, black pepper, camphor, eucalyptus, marjoram, melissa, peppermint, rosemary
Colic   benzoin, bergamot, black pepper, camomile, camphor, cardamon, clary, fennel, hyssop, juniper, lavender, marjoram, melissa, peppermint
Colitis   black pepper, bergamot, camomile, lavender, neroli, rosemary, ylang-ylang
Conjunctivitis   camomile, lavender, rose (compress)
Constipation   black pepper, camphor, fennel, marjoram, rose
Convulsions   camomile, clary, lavender
Cough   benzoin, black pepper, cardamon, cypress, eucalyptus, frankincense, hyssop, jasmine, juniper, myrrh, peppermint, sandalwood
Cystitis   bergamot, cedarwood, eucalyptus, juniper, lavender, sandalwood
Depression   basil, bergamot, camomile, camphor, clary, geranium, jasmine, lavender, melissa, neroli, patchouli, rose, sandalwood, ylang-ylang
Dermatitis   benzoin, camomile, hyssop, geranium, juniper, lavender, peppermint
Diabetes   eucalyptus, geranium, juniper
Diarrhoea   black pepper, camomile, camphor, cypress, eucalyptus, geranium, lavender, myrrh, neroli, peppermint, rosemary, sandalwood
Diphtheria   bergamot, eucalyptus, lavender
Disinfection (of rooms) bergamot, eucalyptus, juniper, lavender

Dispnoea camphor, hyssop

Dropsy juniper

Dysentery black pepper, camomile, cypress, eucalyptus, melissa

Dysmenorrhoea see *menstruation*

Dyspepsia see *stomach*

Dysuria black pepper, cedarwood, juniper

Earache see *otitis*

Eczema bergamot, camomile, geranium, hyssop, juniper, lavender

Emphysema eucalyptus

Enuresis cypress

Epilepsy basil, lavender, rosemary

Fainting basil, black pepper, camomile, lavender, melissa, peppermint, rosemary

Fevers basil, black pepper, bergamot, camomile, camphor, eucalyptus, hyssop, melissa, peppermint

intermittent: basil, bergamot, black pepper, camomile, eucalyptus

Fistula (anal) lavender

Flatulence bergamot, black pepper, camomile, camphor, cardamon, clary, fennel, hyssop, juniper, lavender, marjoram, myrrh, peppermint, rosemary

Frigidity see *impotence*

Gall bladder

cholecystitis: rose, rosemary

stones: bergamot, eucalyptus, lavender, peppermint, rosemary

Gastralgia see *stomach*

Gastritis see *stomach*

Genital erethism marjoram

Gingivitis camomile, myrrh

Glossitis bergamot, geranium

Gonorrhoea bergamot, cedarwood, eucalyptus, frankincense, lavender, sandalwood

Gout basil, benzoin, camphor, fennel, juniper, rosemary

Haemorrhage	cypress, eucalyptus, frankincense, geranium, rose
Haemorrhoids	cypress, frankincense, juniper, myrrh
Halitosis	bergamot, cardamon, lavender, peppermint
Hay fever	eucalyptus?, rose (also see *allergies*)
Headache	camomile, cardamon, lavender, marjoram, peppermint, rose, rosemary
Heart	
heart failure:	camphor
palpitations:	lavender, melissa, neroli, peppermint, rosemary, ylang-ylang
Heartburn	see *stomach*
Herpes	bergamot, eucalyptus
Hiccough	see *stomach*
Hypercholesterolaemia	rosemary
Hyperglycaemia	eucalyptus
Hyperpnoea	ylang-ylang
Hypertension	see *circulation*
Hypotension	see *circulation*
Hysteria	basil, camomile, camphor, clary, hyssop, lavender, marjoram, neroli, peppermint, rosemary
Impotence	clary, jasmine, rose, ylang-ylang
Indigestion	see *stomach* (dyspepsia)
Influenza	black pepper, cypress, eucalyptus, hyssop, lavender, peppermint, rosemary
Insomnia	basil, camphor, camomile, lavender, marjoram, neroli, rose, sandalwood, ylang-ylang. May be due to poor digestion, 'liverishness', or other gastro-intestinal disturbance. May also be due to excess heat in some part of the body, in which case a camomile and rose compress should be applied
Itching	see *pruritis*
Jaundice	see *liver*

Kidney
general: cedarwood, clary, eucalyptus, juniper, sandalwood
nephritis: camomile, eucalyptus
pyelitis: cedarwood, juniper
Laryngitis   benzoin, frankincense, lavender, sandalwood
Leucorrhoea   bergamot, clary, eucalyptus, frankincense, hyssop, juniper, lavender, marjoram, myrrh, rose, rosemary
Lice   see *pediculosis*
Liver
chlorosis: lavender, myrrh, rosemary
cirrhosis: juniper, rosemary
congestion: camomile, cypress, rose, rosemary
hepatitis: rosemary
jaundice: geranium, rosemary
Loss of appetite   see *appetite*
Loss of voice   cypress, lavender
Malarial fever   basil, eucalyptus
Measles   eucalyptus
Memory (weak)   see *mental fatigue*
Menopause   camomile, cypress, fennel
(problems of)
Menorrhagia   see *menstruation*
Menstruation
amenorrhoea: camomile, clary, fennel, hyssop, juniper, myrrh
dysmenorrhoea: camomile, clary, cypress, jasmine, juniper, marjoram, melissa, peppermint, rosemary
irregular: clary, melissa, rose
menorrhagia: cypress rose
scanty: see *amenorrhoea*. Also: basil, lavender, marjoram, melissa, peppermint, rose, rosemary

Mental fatigue
(poor concentration,   basil, cardamon, peppermint,
(weak memory)   rosemary

Migraine	basil, camomile, eucalyptus, lavender, marjoram, melissa, peppermint, rosemary. May be related to nervous disturbance, or digestive disorders (intestinal or hepatic congestion/intoxication)
Nausea	see *stomach*
Nephritis	see *kidney*
Nervous tension (anxiety)	benzoin, bergamot, camomile, camphor, cypress, geranium, jasmine, lavender, marjoram, melissa, neroli, patchouli, rose, sandalwood, ylang-ylang
Nettle rash	see *urticaria*
Neuralgia	camomile, eucalyptus, geranium, peppermint
facial:	camomile, geranium
Neurasthenia	clary, lavender, marjoram,
Nosebleed	cypress, frankincense
Obesity	fennel, juniper, patchouli
Oedema	juniper, patchouli
Oliguria	fennel, juniper, lavender
Ophthalmia	camomile, clary, geranium, rose
Otitis	basil, camomile, hyssop, lavender
Palpitation	see *heart*
Paralysis	basil, lavender, peppermint
Pediculosis (lice)	eucalyptus, geranium, lavender, rosemary
Pneumonia	camphor
Polypus (nasal)	basil
Pregnancy	frankincense, jasmine, melissa, rose
Pruritis (itching)	camomile, cedarwood, jasmine, peppermint (essences must be used in concentrations less than 1% for external use)
vaginal:	bergamot, camomile
Psoriasis	bergamot, lavender
Pyelitis	see *kidney*
Pyorrhoea	cypress, myrrh
Pyrosis	see *stomach*

Quinsy   black pepper, hyssop
Rejuvenation
(general)   frankincense, jasmine, lavender,
                          melissa, myrrh, patchouli, rose
Rheumatism (rheumatoid arthritis)
local: camomile, camphor, eucalyptus,
                          lavender, rosemary
general: benzoin, cypress, eucalpytus, hyssop,
                          juniper, lavender, rosemary
Ringworm   geranium, peppermint
Scabies   bergamot, lavender, peppermint,
                          rosemary
Scarlet fever   eucalyptus
Scrofula   frankincense, hyssop, lavender
Shingles   eucalyptus, geranium, peppermint
Shock   camphor, melissa, neroli, peppermint
Sinusitis   eucalyptus, lavender, peppermint
Skin care
chapped: benzoin, camomile, geranium,
                          patchouli, rose, sandalwood
dry: camomile, geranium, jasmine,
                          lavender, neroli, rose, sandalwood,
                          ylang-ylang
inflamed: camomile, clary, geranium, myrrh,
                          peppermint, rose, sandalwood
mature: benzoin, clary, cypress,
                          frankincense, lavender, myrrh,
                          neroli, patchouli, rose
normal: geranium, jasmine, lavender, neroli,
                          rose
oily: bergamot, camphor, cedarwood,
                          cypress, frankincense, geranium,
                          juniper, lavender, sandalwood,
                          ylang-ylang
sensitive: camomile, jasmine, neroli, rose
Snake bite   lavender
Spermatorrhoea   benzoin, frankincense
Sprains   camphor, eucalyptus, lavender,
                          rosemary
Sterility   geranium, rose
in women: melissa

304

Stomach

dyspepsia (indigestion): basil, bergamot, black pepper, camomile, cardamon, clary, eucalyptus, fennel, frankincense, hyssop, juniper, lavender, marjoram, melissa, myrrh, peppermint, rosemary

gastralgia: camomile, geranium, peppermint

gastritis: camomile

hiccough: basil, fennel, sandalwood

nausea: basil, black pepper, cardamon, fennel, lavender, melissa, peppermint, rose, sandalwood

pyrosis (heartburn): black pepper, cardamon

Stomatitis bergamot, geranium, myrrh

Stones (gall) see *gall bladder*

Stones (urinary) camomile, fennel, geranium, hyssop, juniper

Strangury see *dysuria*

Sunstroke lavender (see also *shock*)

Syphilid hyssop

Teething (infants) camomile

Throat infections clary, eucalyptus, geranium, lavender

Thrush myrrh

Tic marjoram

Tonsillitis (acute) bergamot

Toothache camomile, camphor, peppermint

Trembling see *convulsions* and *palpitations*

Tuberculosis bergamot, camphor, eucalyptus, hyssop, lavender, myrrh, peppermint, sandalwood

Tumours (benign) bergamot, camomile, cedarwood

Typhoid fever eucalyptus, lavender

Ulcers

cornea: lavender

mouth: myrrh

peptic: camomile, geranium

skin: bergamot, camphor, eucalyptus, frankincense, geranium, juniper, lavender, myrrh

varicose: bergamot, lavender

Urinary tract infections see *cystitis*
Urinary stones see *stones*
Urticaria camomile
Vaginitis camomile
Varicose veins
local: cypress
general: non-toxic diet, avoid constipation
Vertigo see *fainting*
Vomiting basil, black pepper, camomile, camphor, cardamon, fennel, lavender, melissa, peppermint, rose, sandalwood
Whooping cough basil, clary, cypress, hyssop, lavender, rosemary
Worms bergamot, camomile, camphor, eucalyptus, fennel, hyssop, lavender, melissa, peppermint
Wounds benzoin, bergamot, camomile, camphor, eucalyptus, frankincense, geranium, hyssop, juniper, lavender, myrrh, patchouli, rosemary

Index of Properties

Please see preface, 159, 319 for advice and information on how to use essential oils.

Adrenal cortex stimulants
     basil, geranium, rosemary

Analgesic (pain-relieving, usually applied locally)
     bergamot, camomile, camphor, eucalyptus, geranium, lavender, marjoram, peppermint, rosemary

Anaphrodisiac (diminishing sexual desire)
     camphor? marjoram

Anthelmintic   see *vermifuge*

Anticonvulsive camomile, clary, lavender

Antidepressant (uplifting, counteracting melancholy)
     basil, bergamot, camomile, camphor, clary, geranium, jasmine, lavender, melissa, neroli, patchouli, rose, sandalwood, ylang-ylang

Antiphlogistic (reducing inflammation, usually associated with vasoconstriction)
     camomile, clary, myrrh, rose

Antiseptic (a substance which inhibits the growth of bacteria; all essences are antiseptic to one or more organisms)
     Some of the most effective, general antiseptics are bergamot, eucalyptus, and juniper

Antispasmodic (relieving smooth muscle spasm)
basil, bergamot, black pepper, camomile, camphor, cardamon, clary, cypress, eucalyptus, fennel, hyssop, juniper, lavender, marjoram, melissa, neroli, peppermint, rose, rosemary, sandalwood

Antisudorific (counteracting perspiration)
cypress

Antitoxic (a substance which counteracts poisoning)
black pepper, juniper, lavender

Aphrodisiac (stimulating sexual desire)
black pepper, cardamon, clary, jasmine, juniper, neroli, patchouli, rose, sandalwood, ylang-ylang

Astringent (binding, causing contraction of the tissues, A local application used to arrest discharges, haemorrhage, seborrhoea, etc.)
cedarwood, cypress, frankincense, geranium, juniper, myrrh, patchouli, peppermint, rose, rosemary, sandalwood

Carminative (easing griping pains and expelling gas from bowels)
basil, benzoin, bergamot, black pepper, camomile, camphor, cardamon, clary, fennel, frankincense, hyssop, juniper, lavender, marjoram, melissa, myrrh, peppermint, rosemary, sandalwood

Cephalic (relating to disorders of the head, especially stimulants of the mind; useful in weak memory, poor concentration)
basil, cardamon, peppermint, rosemary

Cholagogue (stimulating the flow of bile from the gall bladder into the intestine)
camomile, lavender, peppermint, rosemary

Choleretic (stimulating and increasing bile secretion)
lavender, rose, rosemary

Cicatrisant (promoting the formation of scar tissue)
bergamot, camomile, eucalyptus, frankincense, geranium, hyssop, juniper, lavender, patchouli, rosemary

Cordial (a heart tonic)
benzoin, camphor, hyssop, lavender, marjoram, melissa, neroli, peppermint, rose, rosemary

Cytophylactic (stimulating regeneration of cells)
Essences in general, especially lavender and neroli

Deodorant (counteracting body odour)
benzoin, bergamot, clary, cypress, eucalyptus, lavender, neroli, patchouli

Depurative (purifying the blood)
eucalyptus, juniper, rose

Digestive (aiding digestion)
basil, bergamot, black pepper, camomile, cardamon, clary, frankincense, hyssop, marjoram, melissa, neroli, rosemary

Diuretic (producing increased secretion of urine)
benzoin, black pepper, camomile, camphor, cardamon, cedarwood, cypress, eucalyptus, fennel, frankincense, geranium, hyssop, juniper, lavender, rosemary, sandalwood

Emmenagogue (inducing menstruation)
basil, camomile, clary, fennel, hyssop, juniper, lavender, marjoram, myrrh, peppermint, rose, rosemary

Expectorant (facilitating the removal of broncho-pulmonary secretions, especially catarrh)
basil, benzoin, bergamot, cedarwood, eucalyptus, fennel,

Expectorant (*contd.*)   hyssop, marjoram, myrrh, pepper-
                                 mint, sandalwood
Febrifuge (reducing fever)
                                 basil, bergamot, black pepper,
                                 camomile, camphor, eucalyptus,
                                 hyssop, melissa, peppermint
Galactagogue (increasing the flow of milk)
                                 fennel, jasmine
Haemostatic (arresting bleeding, by encouraging coagulation
                      of blood)
                                 geranium, rose
Hepatic (a liver tonic)
                                 camomile, cypress, peppermint,
                                 rose, rosemary
Hypertensor (raising arterial blood pressure)
                                 camphor, hyssop, rosemary
Hypoglycemiant (lowering blood sugar level)
                                 eucalpytus
Hypotensor (lowering arterial blood pressure)
                                 clary, hyssop, lavender, marjoram,
                                 melissa, ylang-ylang
Laxative (promoting bowel evacuation. The action of essences
                      is relatively mild)
                                 black pepper, camphor, fennel,
                                 marjoram, rose
Nervine (having a specific action on the nervous system — a
                      nerve tonic; used for nervous
                      disorders in general)
                                 basil, camomile, clary, hyssop,
                                 juniper, lavender, marjoram,
                                 melissa, peppermint, rosemary
Parturient (promoting and easing labour during childbirth)
                                 jasmine, lavender
Rubefacient (local stimulant of circulation, causing redness of
                      skin)
                                 black pepper, camphor, eucalyptus,
                                 juniper, rosemary
Sedative (a nervine having a predominantly calming effect
                      in normal doses)
                                 benzoin, bergamot, camomile,
                                 camphor, cedarwood, clary,

Sedative (*contd.*)   cypress, frankincense, geranium,
hyssop, jasmine, juniper, lavender,
marjoram, melissa, myrrh, neroli,
patchouli, rose, sandalwood, ylang-
ylang

Splenetic (a tonic of the spleen)
black pepper, camomile, fennel,
lavender, rose

Stimulant (having a general, predominantly exciting action on
the body)
black pepper, camphor, eucalyptus,
peppermint, rosemary

Stimulants of the circulation: benzoin, black pepper,
camphor, juniper, rosemary

Stimulants of leucocytosis: all essences, especially: bergamot,
camomile, lavender

Stomachic (a tonic of the stomach, used in stomach disorders
generally)
basil, black pepper, camomile,
clary, fennel, juniper, melissa,
myrrh, peppermint, rose, rosemary

Sudorific (inducing perspiration)
basil, camomile, camphor, hyssop,
juniper, lavender, melissa,
peppermint, rosemary

Tonic (giving tone to the body generally, or specifically to
one area; mildly invigorating)
basil, black pepper, camomile,
cardamon, clary, fennel,
frankincense, geranium, hyssop,
jasmine, juniper, lavender,
marjoram, melissa, myrrh, neroli,
patchouli, rose, sandalwood

Skin tonics   bergamot, camphor, cypress,
geranium, juniper, peppermint,
rose, rosemary

Uterine (a tonic of the uterus)
clary, frankincense, jasmine,
melissa, myrrh, rose

Vasoconstrictor (a local application causing constriction of
capillaries)

Vasoconstrictor (*contd.*)   camomile, cypress, peppermint
general (causing systematic vasoconstriction):
                              camphor
Vermifuge (expelling or eliminating intestinal worms)
                              bergamot, camomile, camphor,
                              eucalyptus, fennel, hyssop,
                              lavender, melissa, peppermint
Vulnerary (an agent applied externally, which heals cuts,
                              sores, or other open wounds)
                              benzoin, bergamot, camomile,
                              camphor, eucalyptus, frankincense,
                              geranium, hyssop, juniper,
                              lavender, myrrh, rosemary

Bibliography

The books are classified in chronological order, most of them under the date of original publication. Dates in brackets refer to the edition actually consulted. The thirteenth- and fifteenth-century books are untitled and anonymous, and I have given the library reference number. They can all be found in the library of Trinity College, Cambridge.

Naturally there are many other works which have influenced me, or have provided information on which I have drawn, but I hope to have given credit to the most important. If I have inadvertently omitted anything of note, my humble apologies to the author.

c. 2650BC	*The Yellow Emperor's Classic of Internal Medicine* (translated by Ilza Veith in 1949)
Sometime AD	The Holy Bible
13th century	A medical work in French prose apparently based on the *Chirurgia* of Roger of Salerno (MS 0.1.20)
15th century	MSS 0.1.13; 0.1.57; 0.7.20; 0.8.35; R. 14.32: *An Herbal* (Trinity College, Cambridge)
1525	*Here begynnyth a newe mater, the wiche sheweth and treateth of ye vertues and proprytes of herbes the wiche is called an Herball* (published by Rycharde Banckes, London)
1527	*The Vertuose boke of Distyllacyon of the waters of all maner of Herbes*, Hieronymus Braunschweig (translated from the Dutch by Laurence Andrewe, and published in 1517)

BIBLIOGRAPHY

1633	*The Herball or Generall Historie of Plantes. Gathered by John Gerarde of London Master in Chirurgerie Very much Enlarged and Amended by Thomas Johnson Citizen and Apothecarye of London*, John Gerarde
1652	*The English Physitian, or an Astrologo-physical discourse of the vulgar herbs of this nation. Being a compleat method of physick, whereby a man may preserve his body in health; or cure himself, being sick*, Nicholas Culpeper (also later, enlarged editions, *Culpeper's British Herbal* (1805) etc.)
1660	*ARTS Master-Piece or the beautifying part of PHYSICK. Whereby all defects of nature in both sexes are amended, age renewed, Youth continued, & All imperfections fairly remedied. With many the most approved physical experiments, so far discovered, that every man may be his own apothecary*, Nicholas Culpeper
1722	*Botanicum Officinale; or a compendious HERBAL Giving An account of all such PLANTS as are now used in the Practice of PHYSICK with their Descriptions and Virtues*, Joseph Miller
1865	*The Book of Perfumes*, Eugene Rimmel
1882	*Elements of Pharmacy, Materia Medica and Therapeutics*, William Whitla, MD
1891	*Piesse's Art of Perfumery*, Charles H. Piesse
1907 (1971)	**Potter's New Cyclopaedia*, R. C. Wren
1918 (1973)	*The Herbalist*, Joseph E. Meyer
1922 (1972)	*The Old English Herbals*, Eleanour Sinclair Rohde
1923	*Aromatics and the Soul*, Daniel McKenzie
1927	*The Mystery and Lure of Perfume*, C. J. S. Thompson
1928	*Aromathérapie*, René-Maurice Gattefossé
1931 (1971)	*A Modern Herbal*, Mrs M. Grieve
1931	**Heal Thyself*, Edward Bach
1937 (1973)	**The Gospel of Peace of Jesus Christ*, The Disciple John
1937	**Fragrant and Radiant Symphony*, Roland Hunt
1939	*Les Produits aromatiques utilisés en pharmacie*, Albert Couvreur
1949	*Technique of Beauty Products*, R. M. Gattefossé and Dr H. Jonquières

*Published by The C. W. Daniel Company Ltd., Saffron Walden, Essex.

BIBLIOGRAPHY

1963	*Die physiologischen und pharmakologischen wirkungen der atherischen ole, reichstoffe und verwandten produkte*, Arno Müller
1964	*The Secret of Life and Youth*, Marguerite Maury (translated from *Le Capital Jeunesse*, pub. 1961)
	*Aromathérapie, Dr Jean Valnet
	The Aquarian Gospel of Jesus the Christ, Levi
1966	*Let's Get Well*, Adelle Davis
	Nature's Medicines, Richard Lucas
1967	*Ayurveda for You*, Dr Chandrashekhar
1970	*Odours*, R. W. Moncrieff
1971	*Back to Eden*, Jethro Kloss
	Diet for a Small Planet, Frances Moore Lappé
1972	*Phytothérapie*, Dr Jean Valnet
	A History of Scent, Roy Genders
	Of Men and Plants, Maurice Mességué
1973	*The Magic of Perfume*, Eric Maple
	Supernature, Lyall Watson
	The Secret Life of Plants, Peter Tompkins and Christopher Bird
	Acupuncture, Marc Duke
	Chinese Medicinal Herbs, translated and edited by F. Porter Smith, MD and G. A. Stuart, MD (based on great Chinese teatise known as the *Pên T'sao*, published in 1578 by Li Shih-Chên)
1974	*The Kirlian Aura*, Stanley Krippner and Daniel Rubin
1985	*The Essential Oil Safety Data Manual*, Robert Tisserand

*Published by The C. W. Daniel Company Ltd., Saffron Walden, Essex.

Bibliography (Articles)

Amoore, J.E. Nature 1967, 216, 1084 – 87
Appel, Louis. Amer. Perfum. Cosmet. 1969, 84 (2) 53 – 6
Appel, Louis. Amer. Perfum. Cosmet. 1968, 83 (11) 37 – 47
Arnold, W. Arch. Exptl. Path. Pharm. 1927, 123, 129 – 59
Atanasova-Shopova, S. et al. Izu. Inst. Fisiol. Bulg. Akad. Nauk.
    1970, 13, 67 – 77
Atanasova-Shopova, S. et al. ibid. 89 – 95
Bassiri, T. Soap, Perfum. Cosmet. 1975, 48 (7) 314 – 15
Beets, M.G.J. Parfum. Cosmet. Savon. 1962, 5, 167 – 84
Bergwein, K. Amer. Perfum. & Cosmet. 1968, 83, 41 – 3
Boedecker, Fr. et al. Pharm. Ztg. 1928, 73, 738
Bonn, H.L. Dent. med. Wochschr. 39, 690
Boyd, E.M. et al. Am. J. Medi. Sci. 1946, 211, 602 – 10
Boyd, E.M. et al. J. Pharmacol. Exp. Ther. 1968, 163 (1) 250 – 56
Boyd, E.M. et al. Pharmacol. Res. Commun. 1970, 2 (1) 1 – 16
Braun, H. Fortschr. Therap. 1942, 18, 80
Braun, H. ibid. 83
Caujolle, F. et al. Compt. Rend. Soc. Biol. 1945, 139, 210 – 13
Caujolle, F. et al. ibid. 1109 – 1111
Carvel, L. Compt. Rend. Acad. Sc. 1918, 166, 827 – 29
Clerk, C. et al. Compt. Rend. Soc. Biol. 1934, 116, 864 – 5
Courmont, P. et al. La Parfum. Moderne 1928, 21, 161 – 67
Dandiya, P.C. et al. Can. Pharm. J. Sci. Sect. 1958, 91, 607 – 10
Dandiya, P.C. et al. J. Pharmacol. Exptl. Therap. 1959, 125, 353 – 59
Das, P.K. et al. Arch. Intern. Pharmacodynamie 1962, 135, 167 – 77
Debelmas, A.M. et al. Plant. Med. Phytother. 1967, 1 (1) 23 – 27
Dhalla, N.S. et al. J. Pharm. Sci. 1961, 50, 580 – 82
Dinckler, K. Pharm. Zentralhalle 1936, 77, 281 – 90
Fingerling, G. Landw. Vers. Sta. 67, 253 – 89
Fukuda, T. Arch. Exptl. Path. Pharmakol. 1932, 164, 685 – 94
Fulton, G.P. et al. J. Invest. Dermatol. 1959, 33, 317 – 25

BIBLIOGRAPHY (ARTICLES)

Gattefossé, R.M. La Parfum. Moderne 1937
Gattefossé, R.M. & H.M. Perf. & Ess. Oil Rec. 1954, Dec. 406 – 09
Gatti & Cajola, Riv. Ital. Ess. Prof. 1922, 16 – 23
Gatti & Cajola, ibid. 1923, 133 – 35
Gatti & Cajola, ibid. 1925, 101 – 02
Gatti & Cajola, ibid. 1930, XXI – XXIII
Gatti & Cajola, ibid. 1931, 158 – 60
Gatti & Cajola, ibid. 1932, 108 – 09
Gatti & Cajola, ibid. 1937, 139 – 43
Gatti & Cajola, ibid. 1937, 216 – 22
Gatti & Cajola, ibid. 1937, 248 – 55
Gatti & Cajola, ibid. 1937, 291 – 97
Grisogani, N. Atti. accad. Lincai 1925, (6) 1, 602 – 4
Grochulski, A. et al. Planta Med. 1972, 21 (3) 289 – 92
Gyergyay, F. et al. Histochim. Cytochim. Lipides, Simp. Int. Histol.
    5th Sofia. 1963, 591 – 5
Haginiwa, J. et al. Yakugaku Zasshi 1963, 83, 624 – 8
Hanzlik, P.J. J. Pharmacol. 1923, 20, 463 – 79
Hollander, F. et al. Am. J. Physiol. 1948, 152, 645 – 51
Inaseki, I. et al. Yakugaku Zasshi 1962, 82, 1326 – 8
Jain, S.R. et al. Planta Med. 1971, 20 (2) 118 – 23
Janistyn, H. Amer. Perfumer 1961, Jan. 19 – 21
Jannu, I. et al. Arch. Exptl. Pathol. Pharmacol. 1960, 238, 112 – 13
Jaretzky, R. et al. Arch. Pharm. 1939, 277, 50 – 3
Jenner, P.M. et al. Food Cosmet. Toxicol. 1964, 2 (3) 327 – 43
Jerzy, Maj. et al. Dissertationes Pharm. 1964, 16 (4) 447 – 56
Jordan, A. Biochem. J. 5, 274 – 90
Kar, A. et al. Qual. Plant. Mater. Veg. 1971, 20 (3) 231 – 7
Karlin, M. Farm. Vestn. (Ljubljana) 1968, 19 (5 – 8) 163 – 70
Katz, A.E. Spice Mill 1946, 69, 46 – 51
Kudrzycka-Bieloszabska, F.W. et al. Diss. Pharm. Pharmacol. 1966,
    19 (5) 449 – 54
Macht, D.I. J. Pharmacol. 4, 547 – 52
Macht, D.I. J. Am. Med. Assoc. 1938, 110, 409 – 14
Madan, B.R. et al. Arch. Intern. Pharmacodynamie 1960, 124,
    201 – 11
Marino, V. Ann. igiene 1935, 45, 158 – 76
Maruzella, Jasper et al. J. Am. Pharm. Assoc. 45, 378 – 81
Maruzella, Jasper et al. J. Am. Pharm. Assoc. 1958, 47, 294 – 6
Maruzella, Jasper et al. J. Am. Pharm. Assoc. 1958, 47, 471 – 6
Maruzella, Jasper et al. J. Am. Pharm. Assoc. Sci. Ed. 1960, 49,
    692 – 94
Mashino, K. et al. Sogo Igaka 1953, 10, 805 – 09
Meer, G. et al. Am. Perfumer Aromat. 1960, 75, (11) 38 – 40

BIBLIOGRAPHY (ARTICLES)

Morel, A. et al. Compt. Rend. Soc. Biol. 1922, 86, 933 – 34
Necheles, H. et al. Am. J. Physiol. 1935, 110, 686 – 91
Okanishi, T. Folin Pharmacol. Japon. 1928, 7, 77 – 85
Okazaki, Kanzo et al. J. Pharm. Soc. Japan 1953, 73, 344 – 7
Perutz, A. Med. Klin. 1923, 19, 348 – 50
Piacenti, G. Ann. igiene 1948, 58, 1 – 11
Pusztai, F. et al. Pharmazie 1963, 18, 238 – 41
Ramadan, F.M. et al. Chem. Mikrobiol. Technol. Lebensin. 1972, 2, 51 – 5
Rao, B.G.V. et al. Flavour Ind. 1970, 1, (10) 725 – 29
Rovesti, Paolo. Riv. Ital. Ess. Profum. 1960, 42, 333 – 42
Rovesti, Paolo. Riv. Ital. Ess. Profum. 1962, 44, 266 – 281
Rovesti, Paolo. Fruits 1963, 18, (9) 407 – 11
Rovesti, Paolo. Riv. Ital. Ess. Profum. 1964, 79 – 81
Rovesti, Paolo. Riv. Ital. Ess. Profum. 1971, 53, (5) 251 – 69
Rovesti, Paolo & Gattefossé, H.M. Labo-Pharma, Probl. et. Techn. 1973, 223, 32 – 38
Rovesti, Paolo. Soap, Perfum. and Cosmet. 1973, XLVI (8) 475 – 478
Ruckebusch, Y. La France et ses Parfums 1964, 291 – 98
Sapoznik, H.I. et al. J. Am. Med. Assoc. 1935, 104, 1792 – 4
Short, G.R. Manuf. Chemist 1956 March, 96 – 98
Schweissheimer, W. Parf. Cosmet. Savons 1958, 353 – 56
Shipochliev, T. Vet.-Med. Nauki 1968, 5, (6) 63 – 9
Shipochliev, T. ibid. 5 (10) 87 – 92
Skramlik, E.V. Discovery 1958, 19, 373 – 76
Skramlik, E.V. Pharmazie 1959, 14, 435 – 45
Slavenas, J. Obshch. Zakonomer. Rosta Razu. Rast., Dokl. Nauch. Konf. Vilynus 1963, 313 – 38
Some, Y. et al. Tohoku J. Exptl. Med. 1937, 30, 540 – 45
Stickney, J.C. Proc. Soc. Exptl. Biol. Med. 1943, 52, 274 – 75
Valette, G. Compt. Rend. Soc. Biol. 1945, 139, 904 – 6
Vasileva, E.N. et al. Farmakol. Toxicol. (Moscow) 1972, 35 (3) 312 – 15
Vichkanova, S.A. et al. Farmakol. Toxicol. (Moscow) 1973, 36 (3) 339 – 41
Vedibeda, D.K. Gigiena i Sant. 1958, 23, (8) 80
Wagner, H., et al. Dent. Apoth.-Ztg. 1973, 113 (30) 1159 – 66
Winter, A.G. Planta Med. 1958, 6, 306 – 13
Wright, R.H. J. Appl. Chem. 1954, 4, 611 – 21
Wright, R.H. et al. Chem. & Ind. 1956, 973 – 77
Zavarzin, G.M. et al. Vop. Med. Feor., Klin Prakt. Kurottnogo Lech. 1971, 4, 300 – 02
Zolotov, V.S. Arch. Sci. biol. 1931, 31, 314 – 21
Zondek, B. et al. Biochem. J. 1938, 32, 641 – 45

Recommended Therapeutic Dosages

Age group	No. of drops if given alone	No. of drops if with other oils	Doses per day	Maximum treatment period
Adults (15 +)	3	2	3	3 weeks
10 – 14 years	2	1	3	2 weeks

Important

For most purposes one or two essences will be quite sufficient, and three should be regarded as a maximum.

All essences should be taken in honey water, after food. (See p. 160 regarding honey water). Never take essences undiluted, or on an empty stomach.

Since jasmine, rose absolute, and benzoin are not essential oils their usage should be limited to external applications only.

Courses of Treatment

The treatment periods given above are *maximums*. One week will be sufficient in most cases, and a few days is often adequate when treating acute conditions. In very chronic cases allow two weeks in between courses for every week of treatment given. Beware of using certain essences over long periods — see *chronic toxicity*.

Young Children

It is not advisable to prescribe certain essences internally for children younger than 10 years, unless under professional advice. (An exception may be made for peppermint oil, diluted by honey water, as a home-made 'gripe-water', when 1 drop may be given as a dose.) Children do respond very quickly to aromatherapy, and in all other cases baths, compresses, inhalations or massage oils will achieve a successful result.

Acute Toxicity

Extremely high doses (10 – 20 ml) of certain essential oils can result in poisoning. However, none of the oils discussed in this book, are toxic.

Chronic Toxicity

The prolonged use of some essences, *in abnormally high doses* can result in chronic poisoning and cause tissue degeneration.

Toxicity and Pregnancy

Both types of toxicity can be caused by oils of calamus, pennyroyal, sage (but not clary sage) and wintergreen. These should be avoided altogether. With certain oils there is a very low risk of causing abortion, especially if the dosage or dilution is too high. For this reason it is best to avoid basil, hyssop, myrrh, marjoram and thyme during pregnancy.

Allergic Reaction

In some people (although this is extremely rare) there is an idiosyncratic, or allergic reaction to a particular essence. In these cases a normal therapeutic dose can cause symptoms of intoxication; e.g. eucalyptus oil could produce symptoms affecting the skin and/or the nervous system.

Summary

There is a minimal risk of allergic reaction, and no risk of toxicity if essences are prescribed in the dosages given for no longer than the period of time given.

There is even less risk when using essences externally (diluted to 2 – 3%) but it is not advisable to use higher concentrations over a long period of time. When treating very chronic conditions it may be preferable to use the prescription externally (suitable diluted) although even here it is advisable to limit a single course of treatment to something like ten weeks, for daily applications, and thirty weeks for weekly applications.

Amounts less than those given may always be used (see p. 78).

Training Courses

I do teach aromatherapy, for those who seriously wish to learn the art, and I also run a one-day seminar for lay people. If you are interested in either courses or seminars, please contact me through my publisher, The C. W. Daniel Company Limited, 1 Church Path, Saffron Walden, Essex CB10 1JP, England.

Where to Obtain Essential Oils

Aroma Vera Inc.
P.O. Box 3609
Culver City, CA 90231
(213) 973-4253

All the oils distributed by Aroma Vera are extracted from either wild or organically grown plants. The massage oils are specially blended for specific purposes as are the blends for use in diffusers. They also sell diffusers and books.

The Attar Bazaar
P.O. Box 99
Sidney, NY 13838
(607) 895-6368

Importers of alcohol-free natural perfumes and essential oils from Middle and Near East and India. More than 100 attars— natural perfumes—and all natural skin care products and aromatherapy massage oils. Free catalog.

Aura Cacia
P.O. Box 3157
Santa Rosa, CA 95402
(707) 795-1312

Aura Cacia offers essential oils and has also created a line of wonderfully rich and exotic True Botanical Perfume Essences.

Colin Ingram
207 Bohemian Highway
Freestone, CA 95472
(707) 823-1330

Colin Ingram has been a major supplier of high-quality essential oils to the natural cosmetics industry for over sixteen years and offers a large selection of perfumes and essential oils.

Essentials
R.D.#2 Box 160A
Ghent, NY 12075
(518) 672-4519

Essentials is the cooperatively owned company of the Akwenasa
Community which offers products based on aromatherapy. Their
oil blends are designed to be both aesthetically pleasing and
therapeutically beneficial.

InterNatural
P.O. Box 580
Shaker Street
South Sutton, NH 03273
(603) 927-4776

A leading distributor of personal care products, homeopathic
medicines, Bach Flower Remedies, and products for
aromatherapy.

Leydet Oils
P.O. Box 2354
Fair Oaks, CA 95628
(916) 965-7546

Sells excellent quality, pure essential oils as well as aromatic diffu-
sors and books. Also provides classes and a wide range of special
blends, hydrosols, and carrier oils. Write for brochure.

Original Swiss Aromatics
P.O. Box 606
San Rafael, CA 94915
(415) 459-3998

Offers a wide selection of essential oils which are packaged in air-
tight dropper bottles. It also sells floral waters, face, body, and
massage oils, aromatic diffusers, and books on aromatherapy.

Weleda Inc.
841 South Main Street
P.O. Box 769
Spring Valley, NY 10977
(914) 356-4134

Offers a lovely and comprehensive, full-color catalog of body and massage oils, creams, soaps, herb blends, and toiletries for men, women, and children.

Some of this information was obtained courtesy of East West magazine. For further information write to:

American Aromatherapy Association
P.O. Box 1222
Fair Oaks, CA 95628

AROMATHERAPY WORKBOOK
Marcel Lavabre

A leader in the field of aromatherapy brings his years of experience to this practical handbook, showing how these sensually appealing preparations can benefit both mind and body. Here are instructions for preparing your own essences, and details on more than seventy essential oils — botanical classification, medicinal properties, uses for massage and skin care, and their specific action.

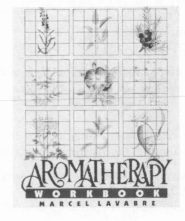

ISBN 0-89281-346-6
$12.95 paperback

THE PRACTICE OF AROMATHERAPY
A Classic Compendium of Plant Medicines and Their Healing Properties
Jean Valnet, M.D.
Edited by Robert Tisserand

One of the world's acknowledged experts in plant medicine, Dr. Valnet details more than forty plants and essences useful in the treatment of illness and the relief of pain, including their history, properties, uses, and methods of application. With more than thirty years of work with plant essences, he shows how this ancient therapy can be an effective adjunct to modern medicine.

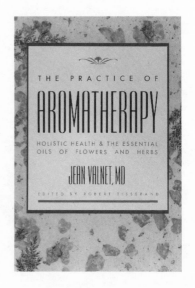

ISBN 0-89281-398-9
$10.95 paperback

"...a fragrant, noninvasive, all-natural means to help achieve well-being." — **Health**

AROMATHERAPY FOR WOMEN
A Practical Guide to Essential Oils for Health and Beauty
MaggieTisserand

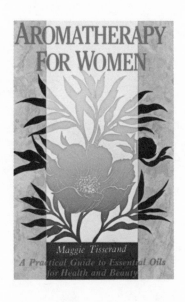

"A very attractive handbook which will lead you into the sensual delights of essential oils and their usefulness."
–Health World

This easy-to-use guide offers an introduction to the many uses of aromatherapy at home, with an emphasis on remedies for women and children. Here is a wealth of simple preparations to enhance sensuality, improve appearance, and alleviate health problems.

ISBN 0-89281-244-3
$6.95 paperback

These and other Inner Traditions/Healing Arts Press titles are available at many fine bookstores or, to order direct, send a check or money order for the total amount, plus $2.00 shipping and handling for the first book and $1.00 for each additional book, to:

Inner Traditions/Healing Arts Press
One Park Street
Rochester, VT 05767

A complete catalog of books is
available on request.